The
New Way
to Live with
Diabetes

The
New Way
to Live with
Diabetes

A COMPLETE GUIDE

by Charles Weller, M.D.,
and Brian Richard Boylan

Illustrated by Howard S. Friedman

DOUBLEDAY & COMPANY, INC.
GARDEN CITY, NEW YORK
1966

Library of Congress Catalog Card Number 66–12225
Copyright © 1966 by
Dr. Charles Weller and Brian Richard Boylan
All Rights Reserved
Printed in the United States of America
First Edition

The authors wish to thank Dr.
Leo Krall of the Joslin Clinic, Boston, Mass., for the many helpful
suggestions he has made.

CONTENTS

PREFACE

Diabetes is an unorthodox disease, a medical nonconformist. It refuses to abide by the convenient rules of conduct established for most of man's other major diseases. Diabetes strikes anyone, anywhere, any time. Even today, thousands of years after it was first observed, diabetes continues to thumb its nose at all attempts to place it in a rigid category.

One of man's deadliest enemies, diabetes is a fascinating disease. Its manifestations are complex; symptoms appear and disappear without warning, and diabetes continues to spread throughout the population—despite the availability of excellent methods and drugs for controlling it. Thus the disease holds a peculiar fascination for its victims, many of whom know as much about its history and causes as their physicians.

The progress against diabetes has been remarkable during this century, yet the disease itself refuses to take note. Each year physicians detect seventy-five thousand new cases of diabetes, but almost as many develop it unknown to themselves or their doctors. The number of unknown diabetics is estimated to parallel roughly the number of confirmed cases. Thus in 1950 there were more than two million known and unknown diabetics, and by 1964 that figure had jumped to four million. However, newer and faster methods of diabetes detection, as well as increased public education, should cut down somewhat on the numbers of unknown diabetics during the next ten years.

The combination of a controllable disease which is still the seventh leading cause of death produces the paradox of diabetes. Why is diabetes still a lethal disease if it is controllable? The answer might be found in the statistics just mentioned. Half of all the diabetics in the United States are undetected; and since survival depends on proper treatment, it is reasonable to classify this undetected half of the diabetic population as in serious trouble. People will continue to suffer from diabetes unnecessarily, simply because they did not recognize the cardinal symptoms and get to a doctor for prompt treatment.

Today's diabetic whose disease is under medical control lives comfortably, with a minimum of inconvenience—a sharp difference from the patient's lot two generations ago. Recent advances in processing and packaging of foods have liberated the diabetic from the restricted diets and mealtime unpleasantness of the past. Although he must still be vigilant about his diet, the patient today generally can eat most of the foods he enjoys without endangering his health.

This book is based on a new theory that diabetes is not one disease, as men have long believed, but rather a group of similar diseases which exhibit different symptoms and require different treatments. Three types of diabetes are discussed separately along with the problems and medical management of each type. The book is organized to provide general information for all diabetics, as well as detailed, specific information for each type. Although physicians recognize that diabetes is not one but several diseases, many patients and potential diabetics may not. It is with the hope of clearly separating the three types and thus providing all diabetics with increased knowledge about their diseases that this book is written. Diabetes permits no secrets; the patient must know almost as much as his physician about his disease. The more he knows, the happier his life will be and the better he can care for his disease.

PART I

The Nature of
Diabetes

CHAPTER 1

Diabetes Today

*Diabetes mellitus** is a chronic or long-term disease resulting from the body's inability to use certain basic elements of everyday food, especially starches and sugars. Often the pancreas fails to produce enough of the hormone insulin, and abnormal amounts of sugar accumulate in the blood and the urine. If untreated, this condition can have serious consequences. Poisons in the blood bombard the brain, producing coma and ultimately death. Although diabetes cannot be cured, it can be effectively subdued and controlled by close medical supervision, proper diet, and drugs.

HISTORY OF DIABETES

Diabetes is almost as old as man. The earliest recorded descriptions of his diseases point to the mysterious illness which carried off men and women in their prime. This could not have been heart disease or cancer (today's mightiest killers), which primitive man would have considered afflictions of extreme old age, since anyone over thirty in those days was a patriarch. It is also possible to rule out the more obvious killers such as infectious diseases and plague, because they strike swiftly and leave telltale signs.

* This is unlike a similarly named but completely different disease, *diabetes insipidus,* which is caused by a defect of the pituitary gland and is treated in a different manner with other drugs. The disease this book is concerned with is *diabetes mellitus.*

This strange malady gripped the hardiest warriors as well as women and children, inexorably sapping strength without any physical disfigurement. The only warning signs such prehistoric diabetics might have had would have been excessive hunger and thirst and frequent urination. These symptoms might have appeared gradually or all at once. However, they ultimately would lead to a general loss of energy and strength, physical debilitation, coma and death. The process could be dragged out for years, but it seems more likely that diabetes struck swiftly in early man.

Throughout the centuries of man's struggle toward knowledge, he was prey to what might have been diabetes. But tracing any disease back through history is no easy task, because primitive man took many thousands of years to sort out and dispose of the cobwebs of superstition and theology that had impeded his thinking. Clinical observation, which is so essential to tracing and identifying a disease, was usually replaced by subjective interpretation of illness as a manifestation of divine wrath. Primitive man rarely observed disease objectively enough to give an accurate account of its symptoms and course. Thus, little valuable information about diabetes was obtained until the time of the Romans.

The Roman era saw the first scientific study of the disease, which Roman physicians called *diabetes,* which means *to pass through,* because they thought the frequent urination was due to weak kidneys. The Romans were intrigued by the disease, and soon they were able to present the first accurate description of diabetes.

Unfortunately, interest in diabetes (as well as in

other areas of science) died with the Romans, who had reached a pinnacle of medical knowledge unequaled through the subsequent centuries of the Dark Ages. As Christianity swept through Europe, Roman civilization crumbled, and with it all the scientific knowledge it had acquired. Men were taught (and believed) that they had but a few years left to live before everyone would go to heaven or hell. Therefore, medieval theologians argued convincingly, why should man worry himself about such worldly trivialities as health, disease, or medicine? A man could profit his soul more by studying dogma than by wondering why God had arranged to punish sinners with sickness and death.

This attitude set the tone of learning for several centuries. The healing art degenerated into guesswork since physicians could only surmise about the interior of the human body. Autopsy and dissection were expressly prohibited by ecclesiastical fiat, and the sciences of anatomy and pathology were kept at bay for hundreds of years.

During the Renaissance, however, intelligent men shook themselves free of enforced ignorance. But many centuries had passed between the fall of Rome and Leonardo da Vinci's first anatomical drawings at the beginning of this reawakening of interest in the arts and sciences. Inquisitive men had to forget the intellectual rubbish of the Dark Ages and start afresh. It wasn't until the seventeenth century that a significant breakthrough was achieved when an Oxford physician named Willis demonstrated that diabetes is accompanied by sugar in the urine.

From this point until the twentieth century, the

charting of diabetes proceeded at an unspectacular but steady pace. Watching helplessly as their patients wasted slowly or died suddenly, physicians guessed that some defect in the pancreas prevented the proper chemical breakdown of sugar, permitting it instead to accumulate in the blood. They knew that death resulted from kidney failure or coma, but they knew of no herb or drug capable of reversing the disease once it had started. By the dawn of the twentieth century, scientists suspected that diabetes was probably hereditary rather than infectious, that it very likely flourished in the same families but was not spread by germs. But the riddle of how the disease selected its victims and why some of them died immediately while others lingered on for years was compounded by frustration at not being able to stop its progress. In milder cases, elimination of sugar from the diet provided temporary relief.

Then one hot summer night in 1921 in a cramped laboratory at the University of Toronto, two inexperienced young investigators dramatically discovered that an extract from a dog's pancreas, when injected into a diabetic dog, eliminated sugar from the urine and strikingly lowered the blood sugar level. This extract, which they later called insulin, was the result of months of trials and errors by Dr. Frederick G. Banting, a twenty-nine-year-old unsuccessful orthopedic surgeon, and Charles Best, a twenty-two-year-old medical student. Banting and Best had defied established academic pooh-poohing of their theories, and they were able to conduct their experiments only because Banting had pestered the head of the physiology department at the university for permission to use a laboratory and some experimental dogs during the quiet summer months.

After their first success with insulin, the two investigators repeated it again and again before they announced their discovery late the following year. Waves of publicity about the new "cure" for diabetes brought thousands of requests for insulin from doctors and patients throughout the world—before Banting and Best had tested it on humans. This they did, and the results are history.

During the next twenty years physicians realized that while insulin was valuable in keeping many diabetics alive, it seemed to have an adverse effect on other victims of the disease. At first it was thought that some diabetics were allergic to insulin, just as some today are allergic to certain antibiotics. However, it became apparent that insulin was actually speeding up complications in some diabetics. The belief that insulin was only a partial answer to diabetes led to the development by Dr. Auguste Loubatières in France in 1942 of oral drugs which lowered blood sugar levels but did not stimulate other symptoms. These drugs, called the oral hypoglycemic agents,* did not join insulin in the clinical repertoire until 1956, when tolbutamide (*Orinase*) was introduced in the U.S.

While many diabetics were liberated from the annoyance of the daily insulin injections, insulin therapy was clearly indicated for others. There is no *one* treatment for diabetes, any more than a one-size suit or a one-size hat would fit all people. The fact that it is possible to treat some forms of diabe-

---

* Oral hypoglycemic agent: any medicine which, when swallowed, lowers the amount of sugar in the blood.

tes by pill rather than by injection often confuses new diabetics and their families. A patient who learns for the first time that he has diabetes may know another diabetic who is being treated orally. Therefore if the first patient is told he must inject insulin every day, he is likely to think that his doctor hasn't heard of the pills yet. This response is a trivial but common result of inadequate knowledge about the disease and its management.

Fortunately, the majority of the diabetic population today can be helped by pills. This group includes those who have developed the disease after reaching maturity (and usually middle age). Those who contract it during childhood or teens usually require insulin for the remainder of their lives.

But regardless of whether a needle or a pill is used to control diabetes today, either is superior to the misery and disability which were the plight of the diabetic before 1921. Faithful use of medication, proper adherence to dietary restrictions, and regular visits to the family physician are the primary requirements for a full, normal, reasonably comfortable life.

CARDINAL SYMPTOMS

The cardinal symptoms of diabetes are three: increased thirst and appetite, and frequent urination. Secondary symptoms include weight loss, itchy skin, frequent fatigue, cuts and bruises which heal slowly, changes in vision, pains or cramps in the fingers or toes, drowsiness, and sugar in the urine. Although one can have diabetes without any of these symptoms being present, they serve as indications that something *might* be wrong, and consultation with a physician is advisable.

TYPES OF DIABETES

What is the physical condition of the typical diabetic? Since the disease refuses to be stereotyped in its manifestations, it is useful to describe three general categories of diabetes, Types A, B, and AB.

Type A, insulin-dependent diabetes. A thin man of eighteen years of age has been experiencing the cardinal symptoms of frequent urination and excessive hunger and thirst for about six weeks before seeing his physician. He had been feeling run-down and has recently broken out with boils. A family history reveals that his grandfather as well as other relatives had diabetes. This young man is insulin-dependent and will remain so all his life. Without insulin, his life expectancy is only a few months. In exchange for the slight discomfort of daily injections, this youth can lead a full life—which his grandfather could not. However, he must be especially careful of his diet, and must see his physician regularly in order to avoid complications of the disease.

Another manifestation of Type A can be seen in children. A seven-year-old has been dragging around the house and his teacher has complained that he frequently dozes during her inspiring lectures. His primary interest at school seems to be getting to the water fountain as often as possible, and his fellow pupils razz him about his constant need to drain his bladder. Although he is thin and sallow in appearance, his father is convinced that the boy is feeding his supper to the family dog, for he can't get enough to eat or drink. His mother brings him to the doctor's office after he has had symptoms for only a week; his disease is the rapid-onset variety. This boy, like the eighteen-year-old described above, is insulin-dependent and will remain so the rest of his life. Unfortunately, he is not sufficiently mature to understand the gravity of his disease, and thus the burden of watching his diet, testing his urine and supervising daily injections falls on his parents, who must learn as much about diabetes as if they had the disease themselves.

Type B, overweight diabetes. A fifty-five-year-old married woman has been overweight for several months, and lately she has been complaining that she "doesn't feel well." She is easily fatigued and recently suffered a severe emotional shock when her father died suddenly. When she finally visits her doctor, he discovers from her medical history that her children have all weighed ten pounds or more at birth. Close questioning reveals that she has recently been suffering a burning vaginal itch. A urinalysis shows sugar in her urine and confirms that she has the most common type of diabetes, one shared by 80 per cent of the total diseased population. Her diabetes is not due to an insulin deficiency, but rather to anti-insulin factors which prevent the insulin from being active. Therefore she can be controlled with oral drugs. In her case insulin definitely should not be used since it would cause her to gain unnecessary and undesirable weight. Loss of weight would effectively eliminate many of the serious symptoms of her disease.

Type AB, stress diabetes. A thirty-year-old man of normal weight is in good physical health except during emotional stress. When under unusual strain, he exhibits the cardinal symptoms of hunger, thirst, and urination. If he is sufficiently prudent to tell his doctor about these symptoms, his rather mild diabetes can be checked. Although he may need insulin only in times of severe stress, he will have to see his physician frequently, since his type of diabetes is unpredictable. This is necessary because such individuals often do not realize they are under strain and need insulin. If they neglect or ignore the symptoms, they can change to the totally insulin-dependent category.

Each of these patients represents one aspect of the disease. Although they are composites, they are sufficiently typical to indicate the different ways in which diabetes strikes different individuals. It is not a disease of old age nor is it restricted to children. It visits the fat as well as the thin, women as well as men. However, there are certain trends in diabetes which have become apparent in recent years.

CHAPTER 2

Who Gets Diabetes?

Anyone with a history of diabetes in the family or with the symptoms of the disease will logically ask: Who gets diabetes? The answer is succinct: Anyone. Diabetes is a democratic disease. It does not discriminate by age, nationality, race, or physique. In considering diabetes, it is essential to discard the rumors and the legends.

Diabetes may strike immediately after birth or it can linger until middle age or later. However, statistics indicate that today diabetes shows a slight preference for women and middle-aged persons. In the United States the disease is most prevalent in the northeastern states.

Despite its freewheeling tendencies, diabetes has been known long enough to enable investigators to fit it into certain general categories. For example, the most common form of the disease (Type B—overweight diabetes) is distinctly fond of fat folks. If a middle-aged person is overweight, the chances of his coming down with diabetes are greatly enhanced.

Were the American bookie to forsake the ponies and direct his energies to laying odds on more tangible variables such as disease (as do the insurance companies), he would be willing to establish a fifty-to-one chance on one's getting diabetes. Simplified, this means that out of every hundred nondiabetics at least two and probably four of them would develop the disease in the future.

Although it is impossible for anyone but a physi-

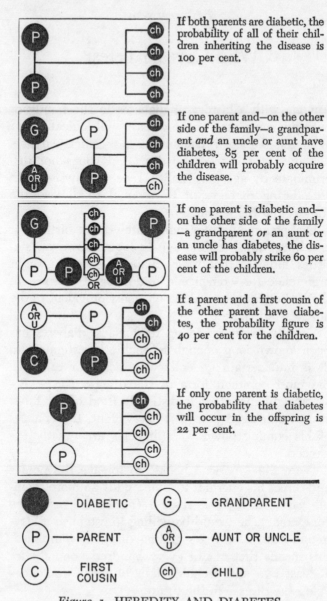

If both parents are diabetic, the probability of all of their children inheriting the disease is 100 per cent.

If one parent and—on the other side of the family—a grandparent *and* an uncle or aunt have diabetes, 85 per cent of the children will probably acquire the disease.

If one parent is diabetic and—on the other side of the family —a grandparent *or* an aunt or an uncle has diabetes, the disease will probably strike 60 per cent of the children.

If a parent and a first cousin of the other parent have diabetes, the probability figure is 40 per cent for the children.

If only one parent is diabetic, the probability that diabetes will occur in the offspring is 22 per cent.

- ● — DIABETIC
- (P) — PARENT
- (C) — FIRST COUSIN
- (G) — GRANDPARENT
- (A OR U) — AUNT OR UNCLE
- (ch) — CHILD

Figure 1. HEREDITY AND DIABETES

cian to determine whether diabetes is present, the following statistical categories should give an indication of a person's chances. Anyone who falls into one or more of these and has the slightest suspicion of any warning symptoms should see his doctor.

FAMILY HISTORY

One of the best predispositions is a family history of diabetes. If genealogical records are sufficiently accurate to include reports of diabetes among various relatives, that is strong evidence for a chat with the doctor. Diabetes occurs five times more often among those with family histories of the disease than among those with no afflicted relatives. The difficulty with tracing hereditary diabetes is that although the disease may have been present in one's ancestors, they often died of other causes before it became manifest. But since diabetes definitely transmits itself from parents to children through generations, any family history deserves serious consideration.

OVERWEIGHT

Another dangerous predisposition is obesity. Four out of five diabetics are overweight before manifesting actual symptoms of diabetes. Obesity is considered by many investigators to be second only to heredity as the most responsible factor in development of the disease.

OVER FORTY

Although diabetes is seen in all age groups (and it is most critical during childhood), it is ten times more common in patients over forty than it is in those under twenty. Perhaps the explanation for this is that the most common form of the disease, Type B, seems to be related to overweight—a problem which is often enhanced by the metabolic changes and generally sedentary life of men and women as they leave physical youth. This, however, is only a theory, and there may be specific physiological mechanisms which stimulate the appearance of diabetes in middle age.

HIGHER INCIDENCE AMONG WOMEN

Two out of three diabetics are women, and more of them are married or have been married than are single. And of married women who contract the disease, the most prevalent are those who have given birth to several children of ten pounds or more. Again, this is a statistical fact that cannot be blamed on any specific factor. One theory is that pregnancy produces certain glandular changes which might predispose a woman to diabetes. Another is that menopause affects the glands adversely and hastens the onset of diabetes. An emotional/psychological view is that being a housewife produces peculiar stresses and tensions. This concept is supported by the tendency of married women to eat more than their systems require.

Like heart diseases, diabetes is much more common among sedentary, inactive people than among those who lead vigorous lives.

Much of the determination about who gets diabetes is based on statistics rather than on factual evidence of physiological disorders. This entire area of investigation will remain one of baffling conjecture until the exact causes of the disease are known.

CHAPTER 3

Diagnosis of Diabetes

Although there has been much emphasis on a family doctor's diagnosis and treatment of diabetes, this emphasis may be somewhat misleading. Diabetes, unlike most other ailments, is patient-managed rather than physician-managed. The doctor determines that the disease is present and how it can best be treated, but the rest is up to the patient. He must learn as much as he can about his disease, and he must understand the symptoms, complications, and proper therapy for all aspects of diabetes. The physician can only guide; he cannot save the patient. The patient's health depends on his own knowledge and understanding of his physical condition. Therefore, good rapport between physician and patient is essential. A remote or disinterested attitude on the part of either can be disastrous, even fatal. Frequent physical examinations are as important as the various tests that the patient himself must carry out. There can be no cheating on diet or skimping on medication. Shortcuts in diabetes lead only to the hospital.

TESTS FOR DIABETES

There are two key tests which the physician performs in his office once he suspects that diabetes may be present. The first is a blood sugar test, a chemical procedure which involves analysis of the percentage of sugar in the blood. For this, he will draw half a tablespoon—two cubic centimeters (or cc's)—of blood from the arm or the finger: a painless, brief test.

The other step in diagnosing diabetes is a sugar tolerance test, which requires several hours of the patient's time, yet it is also painless. The patient reports to the doctor's office early in the morning, without having eaten anything since the previous midnight. The patient swallows a sweet-tasting solution which contains a measured amount of glucose, and his blood is drawn in tiny amounts every hour for several hours to determine whether there is an abnormal degree of sugar in the blood. A urine specimen will be analyzed for the presence of sugar at the same times.

BORDERLINE DIABETES

If the results of these tests indicate the presence of diabetes, the physician will then classify as to type and variabilities, and prescribe medication and diet. However, there is also the chance that the disease may be borderline, and therefore the patient is not a true candidate for either needle or oral therapy at first. If this is the case, it will be necessary to keep in close touch with the doctor so that he can observe the progress of the symptoms and determine whether they represent true diabetes.

PART II

Control of
Diabetes

CHAPTER 4

Diet

To most persons diet means an attempt to lose weight by not eating their favorite foods. Despite reassuring essays in the women's magazines ("gee whiz" medicine), dieting is not fun, nor is it easy. A serious diet usually deprives the patient of foods and beverages he profoundly enjoys, in order to get his body weight down to its proper level.

There are two distinct types of diet, one to lower weight by *restricting* caloric intake, and the other to control metabolism by *regulating* amounts of food. The diabetic must adhere to the second diet at all times, and, if overweight, he may also have to follow the first. One of the few common denominators for all types of diabetes is proper diet to keep the disease under good control.

A diabetic's diet must accomplish many purposes, most important of which is compensating for basic flaws in his metabolism—the process by which the body digests, dissolves, and simplifies food, transforming it into human tissue and energy.

A simple weight-reducing diet is not enough for a diabetic, for there are certain foods he must avoid even though they may not increase his weight.

Since each type of diabetes has its own metabolic problems and nutritional needs, this chapter is concerned primarily with general information that is pertinent to all diabetics. For specific advice the individual should consult his physician.

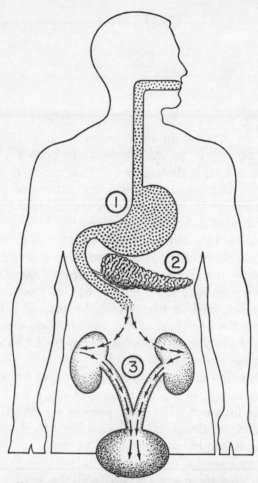

Figure 2. METABOLISM IN DIABETES

Foods and liquids are processed and broken down into fats, proteins, and carbohydrates while in the stomach (**1**). The carbohydrates, however, are not properly absorbed because the pancreas (**2**) fails to secrete enough active insulin to burn up carbohydrates and store them in the liver to supply body tissues with energy. Therefore, the sugar or glucose form of carbohydrate increases excessively in the blood, overflows, and passes through the kidneys (**3**) into the urine.

METABOLISM

To better understand the complexities of diet and diabetes, a brief review of what happens to food once it is swallowed is in order. The body requires three elements from food—carbohydrates for heat and energy, protein for forming blood and muscle tissue, and fat to protect and cover the vital organs.

Carbohydrates, which are of maximum concern to the diabetic, come from sugars and starches (potatoes, bread). These foods are broken down into glucose, which in turn supplies the cells of the body with fuel for heat and energy.

Protein is provided by meat, eggs, and dairy products. Although it is essential to life, protein is no problem in any diet as long as the patient gets enough of it.

Fats, which also must be closely watched by the diabetic, come from such foods as butter, bacon, cheese, milk, cream, and peanuts.

INSULIN

As the glucose enters the bloodstream to carry the heat and energy to the various organs of the body, cells in the pancreas, a gland located just behind the stomach, begins to secrete insulin, a hormone which regulates the amount of glucose, or sugar, in the bloodstream. These cells are called Islets of Langerhans. Too much sugar is dangerous, and too little sugar is equally harmful. When a pancreas is defective and too little insulin is stimulated, the result is insulin-dependent diabetes. If, on the other hand, excess insulin is produced, too much of the energy-

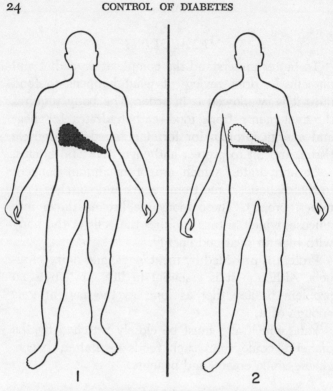

Figure 3. INSULIN AND THE PANCREAS

In the normal individual (**1**) the pancreas has an adequate
supply of insulin, as represented by the dark area. The
insulin-dependent diabetic (**2**) has a pancreas that does not
produce enough insulin.

bearing glucose is burned up, resulting in a condition known as hypoglycemia.

Therefore, the patient with diabetes is suffering
from some unknown, undetectable defect of the
pancreas. The excess sugar in his blood must be controlled either by injecting insulin directly or by taking oral drugs which stimulate the insulin-producing

beta cells of the pancreas to supply enough of the hormone. Because insulin is such a problem, the amount of sugar and starches the diabetic consumes is obviously of great importance in keeping his blood sugar level as close to normal as possible.

One of the first dietary rules for all diabetics is to avoid all sugar and foods containing sugar, such as pastry, candy, soft drinks, etc., and to eat only the permitted portions of spaghetti, potatoes, or other starches. A list of foods to be avoided is given in Appendix C. How much the individual patient can eat of a given food depends on the severity of his disease, his body weight, and a medical evaluation of his nutritional needs. The underweight diabetic will not need to worry about eating fats, although he will have to shun most of the carbohydrates. On the other hand, the overweight middle-aged housewife whose disease is not so severe will have to cut down drastically on both fats and carbohydrates until her weight has reached a proper level.

A second dietary rule is to keep starchy foods evenly distributed among the meals and in the same amounts every day.

It is reasonably easy for the diabetic to learn how to select and prepare the foods which he enjoys yet which conform to the dietary restrictions established by his physician. A detailed knowledge of food chemistry is not necessary.

SOCIAL DINING

The diabetic should know enough about his disease and the effects of foods on it to be able to eat any time and anywhere without embarrassment or worry. He should be able to patronize restaurants and dine out socially, only watching the quantity of foods and avoiding excess carbohydrate.

The quantity of fats and carbohydrates which may be eaten depends to a large extent on how much bulk is present in the food. In other words, a diabetic can eat a large plate of spinach, which contains as much carbohydrate as a tablespoonful of sugar—which itself is specifically prohibited. Spinach is a bulky food, and this bulk slows down the body's absorption of carbohydrate. Bulky foods are also useful when taken simultaneously with high-carbohydrate foods, and physicians recommend a larger quantity of bulk than of high-carbohydrate foods. For example, a patient who eats a plateful of spaghetti should also eat a large green salad to slow down the absorption of carbohydrate from the spaghetti.

THE DIABETIC CHILD'S DIET

Diet is an important factor in the growth of every child, but especially for the diabetic youngster. The mother who throws up her hands in disgust over her child's exclusive interest in milk, cookies, candy, and television is a stereotyped comic figure, for children seem to thrive despite such limited nutrition. However, such a complaint from the mother of a diabetic will not amuse the family doctor. Rather, the diet of the young diabetic is a tricky combination of discipline, clever psychology, and intelligent compromise.

A rough guide for parents of diabetic children is a diet of 1000 calories at age one, with 100 calories added each year until the completion of growth and development (usually between ages sixteen and eighteen). Then, a typical diet consists of 15 calories per pound of ideal body weight. The proportion of carbohydrate, fat, and protein may be close to normal. Interval feedings are urged—that is, equal portions of food taken in midmorning, mid-afternoon, and at bedtime, in addition to regular meals. This interval feeding keeps metabolism at an even level, avoiding sharp peaks of blood sugar levels.

Until recently the dietary restrictions on diabetic children were often unpleasant. Children *had* to eat all the awful-tasting foods, while most of their favorites were arbitrarily outlawed. Much of this reformatory atmosphere has been swept away in recent years. Nutritionists have found that individual attention must be devoted to the patient's likes and dislikes for dieting to succeed. Also, diets for juveniles or young adults now take into consideration the problems of everyday living. For example, many children like to dig into a bowl of ice cream after school, but for years the diabetic youngster had to hang back from this activity. Now, however, parents are told that it is permissible for the child to have ice cream, provided he has the same small amount every day at the same time of day. The diet should remain constant in its food values every day.

The diabetic diet must be adequate to supply the necessary nutrition and energy for the child, but it also should be palatable and sufficiently varied. The diabetic need no longer stand out as a dietary cripple at the family dinner table. He can eat the same basic foods as the rest of the family, while avoiding those which are excessively sweet or to which sugar has been added. The only other restriction is on the amount of food eaten. Thus, the diabetic's eating habits need not exile him to separate meals in the kitchen. It is thoughtful, however, if the family does not tempt him by wolfing down pies and cakes in front of him. A family's sweet tooth has often caused a diabetic some unhappy moments, even provoking him to forsake his diet for the delights of strawberry shortcake. Although giving up sweet desserts may be inconvenient for relatives of a diabetic, they can console themselves with the knowledge that apple pie and fruitcake are not essential to the human diet and, indeed, their excessive consumption can be dangerous.

Dessert can be provided satisfactorily by serving fruits, either fresh or canned (in a water or a sugar-substitute solution), nuts, salad, or gelatin preparations.

The parents of a diabetic child can ignore the "diabetic foods" often found in larger grocery stores. Often the labels are misleading, since most of them contain some sugar. Their chief drawback, however, can be psychological if they convey a false sense of security. There is no food of any kind which a diabetic can eat in unlimited amounts.

CHAPTER 5

Tests for the
Management of Diabetes

Each type of diabetes has its own characteristic symptoms. One can be treated only with insulin, another with oral drugs. But there are some methods of control shared by all diabetics. One is diet, which has already been discussed, but another is urine testing. Every diabetic, regardless of how severe or simple his disease may be, must regularly test his urine. While routine collecting and testing of urine may seem odd to the nondiabetic, the procedure provides both the patient and his physician with an accurate record of the day-to-day management of the disease. Although many patients must examine their urine before each meal and at bedtime, others are on less rigid schedules. Doctors often will reduce the frequency of checks once they have established the disease's pattern in the particular patient. However, patients rarely object to the testing, for it is simple and takes less than one minute.

SUGAR AND ACETONE IN URINE

Two tests can be performed, one for sugar and the other for acetone when sugar is found. Information about sugar and acetone activity in the urine is the doctor's surest indication of how effective his therapy is for that particular patient. (It is impossible to overstress the importance of each patient being treated as a separate individual and not as a member of a group. Although an individual may exhibit most of the common traits of his group, he is likely to have some particular variations from the norm.) The checking of urine is as important to general health of the diabetic as diet, medical examinations, and regular medication. Failure to follow the doctor's instruction about any of these will only result in poor health.

To understand how sugar and acetone get into the urine, it is helpful to visualize the human kidney as a dam. If certain chemicals, including sugar and acetone, accumulate in the bloodstream, the kidney/dam opens, spilling those chemicals into the urine. Acetone is a by-product of sugar in the urine, and the presence of both must be measured accurately. When sugar spills into the urine, it is a sign that diabetes is probably present. When excessive amounts of sugar are lost that way, fats are not completely burned up and ketone bodies (of which acetone is one) accumulate and produce a condition known as ketoacidosis. Because of this chemical chain of events, the physician must know how much sugar is in the urine and whether that sugar is producing acetone. Some patients wonder why such emphasis is placed on both sugar and acetone testing. One major reason is to distinguish between the different types of diabetes. Also, the diabetic and his doctor both have a sharp indicator of when the disease is getting out of control. Acetone in the urine is one such danger sign, for it means that the patient has developed ketoacidosis, which can be tolerated only for a short time by the body. If unchecked, ketoacidosis churns poisons into the blood-stream which rushes them to the brain. When this happens, the patient rapidly goes into diabetic coma, which, if untreated, can be fatal.

Because of the speed with which ketoacidosis can overpower a person, patients themselves are most anxious to make sure that their urine is acetone-free.

The sugar and acetone tests have been refined and simplified in recent years to the point where they are now effortless. Only a generation ago, however, such detection was a complicated, sometimes messy job. For years a preparation known as Bene-dict's solution was the only available method for home testing. This particular test, which has virtu-ally disappeared, required a lot of patience on the part of the patients. The urine was poured into a test tube, mixed with Benedict's solution, and brought to a full boil over a flame until the entire brew changed colors to indicate the amount of sugar in the urine. A pharmacist's skill was needed to pre-vent the mixture from bubbling out of the flask.

CONVENIENT METHODS OF TESTING

Today, fortunately, the diabetic can check his urine for sugar with one of several convenient methods:

Clinitest (Ames Company) is a simplification of the principle behind Benedict's solution, but there is no need of a flame since heat is provided chem-ically by the sodium hydroxide in the tablet con-taining copper salt. Five drops of urine are measured into a test tube (supplied with the test kit), followed by ten drops of water and one Clinitest tablet. As it dissolves, the tablet's internal heat bubbles the mixture. If there is any sugar present, the bubbling heat will cause the mixture to change colors. A blue mixture means no sugar, but if any is present, the solution will first turn green and then, depending on how much sugar is present, it may turn greenish-orange or orange. The color of the liquid is compared with a test chart, which is calibrated by color to indicate the percentage of sugar in the urine. This is essentially a test of *quantity* of sugar.

Clinistix (Ames Company) are strips of paper impregnated with glucose oxidase, an enzyme which reacts to sugar in urine. When the tip of the Clinistix is dipped into the urine and then held in the air for ten seconds, it will change to a purple shade if sugar is present. This is a very accurate test to detect the presence or absence of sugar, rather than the amount. Patients who use Clinistix must also use another test to determine how much sugar is in their urine.

Tes-Tape (Eli Lilly & Co.) determines the quantity as well as the presence of sugar in the urine. A piece of quarter-inch-wide tape is torn from a roll and dipped in the urine specimen. If there is sugar in the urine, the tape will turn a shade of blue, depending on how much there is. By comparing the color of the tape with a chart on the package, the patient can measure the amount of urine in fractions.

Although Tes-Tape and Clinistix tend to be a bit more accurate than Clinitest, the selection of testing materials is governed by personal preference, convenience, and habit. For example, many patients who have been testing their urine for several years with Clinitest seem to prefer it to the newer methods. New diabetics who get started on Tes-Tape, however, generally prefer this method.

Acetone in the urine is as simple to detect as sugar. There are two widely used methods, *Acetest* and *Ketostix* (both manufactured by Ames). A drop of urine is placed on the Acetest tablet, and if the tablet is transformed within one minute to a deep purple, acetone is present in the urine. The Ketostix strip is dipped into urine, held aloft, and examined for any change from its original color to a purple hue, indicating acetone.

A quick reading of the descriptions of these tests might give the newly diagnosed diabetic the impression that he will spend a large part of his life in the bathroom, sampling, testing, and analyzing his urine. This is not true. The tests for acetone and sugar can be performed at convenient times, and the skilled patient can execute them deftly, with no more time, effort, or personal inconvenience than is involved in washing his hands.

For maximum accuracy, patients should not sample the morning's first urine, which has been in the bladder most of the night. Rather, the diabetic should wait approximately twenty minutes after his first urination, and then void a few drops for testing. Just to be extra careful, physicians advise their patients to follow the same procedure when sampling urine before meals and at bedtime. Occasionally the doctor will request a twenty-four-hour specimen for quantitative tests. By analyzing the amount of urine voided in a twenty-four-hour period, the physician can determine precisely how much sugar has

been spilled. The twenty-four-hour specimen requires the patient to collect all his urine during that
period in a single large container. The first urine of
the day is discarded, but from then until the following morning the patient by-passes the customary
toilet facilities in favor of his special collecting jug.
Naturally, some patients are disturbed when asked
to collect a twenty-four-hour specimen. How, they
inquire, are they to drag a large container into the
washroom at work or in public? Since this could be
socially awkward, doctors advise their patients to
collect the specimen on a weekend. After measur-
ing the number of ounces collected, the patient fills
a small specimen bottle with a sample and delivers
it to the doctor's office or laboratory. By noting the
amount passed and by analyzing the sample of that
total urine output, the physician can often resolve
various problems of diagnosis or therapy.

PART III

The Types of Diabetes

CHAPTER 6

Type A:
Insulin-dependent Diabetes

Type A is also known as insulin-dependent diabetes because its victims require insulin throughout their lives. This is the classic form of diabetes, the one most people think of when they hear the name of the disease. Only 15 per cent of all diabetics fall into this category, but it is the most dangerous of the three types, and must be diagnosed, treated, and watched carefully. Type A victims are usually children or young adults, and almost always they are thin. Sexual distribution of the disease, according to the Joslin Clinic in Boston, is divided half and half. The disease generally appears earlier among girls (usually around their tenth birthday) than among boys (thirteenth year) because of earlier female maturity.

The speed with which insulin-dependent diabetes strikes can be seen in the case of Bob M., a seventeen-year-old high school senior. An active athlete, he noticed that recently he was getting unduly tired after a ball game. Also, his thirst seemed to be unquenchable, his appetite had increased noticeably, and he couldn't get through a two-hour game without having to urinate three or four times. His parents smiled tolerantly at these indications that their boy was a typically American, hard-playing, heavily eating and drinking youngster who was forever raiding the icebox between games. When Bob's relatives expressed amazement at his voracious appetite, his parents beamed and murmured the customary proverbs about "a growing boy needs plenty of energy" and "he really burns up food fast."

Bob's football coach, who professionally approved of hearty appetites among his squad, became a bit worried when the boy appeared to be losing weight instead of putting it on. Finally, when Bob had dropped eighteen pounds within two weeks, the coach called his parents.

"Now, don't worry about Sonny," Bob's father reassured the coach. "I know just what's wrong with him—he must be in love with some girl! Yessir, I remember how I couldn't eat or sleep the first time I fell in love."

"That boy's not in love, he's sick," the coach replied. "You'd better get him to a doctor to find out what's wrong. He eats like a horse but he's still losing weight."

Bob's parents questioned him closely about his romantic life and whether he might be worried about his schoolwork or his forthcoming college entrance exams. When it appeared that the boy had no major emotional problems, his father grumblingly yielded to his wife's demands that the boy see a doctor. "He's just an active, growing kid," his father insisted.

The doctor, however, was suspicious as soon as he heard the symptoms. He examined a specimen of Bob's urine and found it full of sugar and acetone. A sample of blood was sent to the laboratory to determine the blood sugar content. While waiting for the lab report, the doctor took an extensive medical history from the boy, including facts about his parents' and relatives' health. The analysis of the sample showed that Bob's blood contained 425 milligrams of sugar. Normal blood sugar contains 80 to 120 milligrams of sugar.

The physician told Bob that he had diabetes and that he would have to be treated for it. Before treatment could begin, however, the doctor needed more specific information about the severity of the boy's disease, his eating habits, exercise needs, emotional problems, and general physical health. He suggested that Bob enter the hospital for a week of observation and testing. As soon as he was admitted to the hospital, nurses, technicians and house physicians joined his doctor in a massive effort to determine Bob's condition as accurately as possible. More blood and urine were taken for additional analysis. The resident physician performed an exhaustive physical examination. The first day, urine was sampled and tested for sugar and acetone every few hours, during which time Bob was given as much water as he wanted to drink. His physician prescribed a special diet which permitted him to have snacks in the middle of the afternoon and at bedtime.

The hospital dietician dropped in for a chat and discussed Bob's likes and dislikes. She described the various types and amounts of foods to be taken, and then reviewed with him the dos and don'ts of dieting. Candy, cake, cookies, pizza, and soft drinks could be taken, occasionally, only in very small quantities. Although he could eat some sugar-based foods, he would have to restrict himself to those items which were on a printed list supplied by the dietician. Most important, the dietician showed Bob how he could eat well at every meal, both at home and in company. By intelligently studying the permissible foods and knowing how much leeway he could grant himself with the questionable foods, Bob need never feel embarrassed or segregated because of his disease.

During his first day in the hospital, Bob was given quick-acting (or regular) insulin every four hours while he was awake. The second day he received an injection of intermediate insulin in the morning, and was told that this was probably the kind of insulin he would be using from then on. The insulin schedule varied for the first few days, with occasional supplemental injections administered when urine tests revealed too much sugar present.

After three days Bob was no longer so hungry or so thirsty as he had recently been. In fact, the food offered him each meal was almost more than he could handle. As he walked around the hospital he felt stronger and did not tire so rapidly as he had before. This was not a sign that he was cured, his doctor warned, but rather an indication that the disease was under control and Bob could resume his normal routine, within certain limitations.

To keep his diabetes under good control at all times, Bob was taught by the nurses how to test his urine for sugar and acetone, and record the results. Since he was, like almost everyone else, a bit frightened of the hypodermic needle, a nurse taught him how to administer the insulin properly by having him practice first with an orange—which offers about the same resistance to the needle as human skin. A few days before he was to go home, Bob started giving himself insulin injections, under the nurse's guidance.

He returned home and to school feeling better than he had for months. His physician told him that his life would be as normal and as long as any of his classmates' provided he watched his diet, regularly tested his urine, administered insulin, and saw his doctor.

Should such a patient neglect any of these measures, one of two consequences can befall him. If his diabetes is severe enough, gross neglect of it might send him into diabetic coma, a life-threatening crisis which requires immediate hospitalization. Should the patient have a milder form of the disease, and if his abuse is not too flagrant, the complications from his neglect might take ten to twenty years to become serious, resulting in disorders of the eyes, blood vessels, or kidneys.

INSULIN DEPENDENCY

Insulin is as much a part of the Type A diabetic's life as his daily shower or morning coffee. Insulin injections are essential, since either his pancreas doesn't produce enough of this vital hormone or his body cannot utilize it effectively. Along with other digestive juices churned out by the pancreas, insulin assists the body to efficiently sort out and dispose of various parts of the food intake, particularly the carbohydrates. In Type A diabetes, when the insulin supply is inadequate, weight, heat, and energy are lost. Insulin, which is produced by tiny cells (the Islets of Langerhans) sprinkled throughout the pancreas, is normally released directly into the bloodstream.

Insulin cannot be taken orally because it is a protein and would be digested, just like meat, by enzymes in the digestive tract. Aware that daily injection of insulin is not the ideal method, scientists once tried sealing the insulin in a coated tablet, which didn't work. Rectal suppositories were also tried and found unsatisfactory. To date, only direct injection is able to carry the insulin into the bloodstream past the chemical barriers which destroy it.

One of the curious inconsistencies of diabetes sometimes is seen immediately after the diagnosis of insulin-dependent diabetes. The first injections of insulin apparently rest the pancreas and the disease seems to subside. That is, the need for insulin often seems to disappear, and the diabetes can be controlled by oral drugs or just by reduction of weight. This hiatus can lull patients into thinking their diabetes is cured, but of course it is not. Usually within a year (but sometimes not for three years) the diabetic's insulin requirements jump once again, and at this point insulin-dependent diabetes has reached its full growth in the individual, and it is not likely to subside again for the rest of his life.

Insulin is commercially available in several types and two strengths. For convenience in administration, most brands are supplied in ampules containing ten cubic centimeters of different concentrations such as U-40 or U-80. These numbers refer to how many units of insulin are contained in each cubic centimeter. This difference in concentration is important to the diabetic, and most insulin syringes are marked with two scales, U-40 and U-80. Common sense urges the patient to make sure that the scale on the syringe corresponds to the strength of insulin he is using.

The three types of insulin are quick-acting, intermediate, and prolonged action. Quick-acting (regular) insulin was also the first available insulin. It acts immediately, but suffers from the disadvantage of not lasting longer than four to six hours. Thus, several injections daily are necessary when regular insulin is used. Intermediate insulin (which is marketed under the trade names of NPH, Lente, and Globin) takes effect two hours after injection and continues for twenty-four hours. Prolonged-action or protamine-zinc insulin doesn't take effect until four hours after injection, but then lasts for twenty-four to thirty-six hours. Protamine-zinc insulin is not widely used today because of the time lag after injection, which necessitates a supplementary dose of regular insulin. Most patients today are controlled on one daily dose of intermediate insulin.

INSULIN INJECTIONS

The shrewd diabetic doesn't pinch pennies or cut corners when purchasing the necessary equipment for insulin injections. Syringes must accurately measure the insulin, and the needles must be sharp, strong, and sterile to avoid painful reactions or infection. An often-used or cheap needle tends to bend easily and could break off in the flesh. Most patients prefer a twenty-five-gauge needle with a length of one-half to five-eighths of an inch. (A quick inspection of a ruler will show that this length is considerably shorter than the needles customarily used by doctors to administer penicillin or other antibiotics.) Recently several companies have introduced a presterilized plastic syringe and needle which are disposable and are usually used only once. This is a boon to the itinerant diabetic who finds sterilizing needles and syringes in his hotel room an inconvenience. The patient opens the sterile pack, fills the syringe with the appropriate amount of insulin, injects it, then disposes of the needle and syringe in the wastebasket.

When using a glass syringe and reusable needle, however, the diabetic must be careful to keep them sterile. The easiest and oldest sterilization method is boiling in water. The needle is attached to the syringe; both are folded in a piece of cloth and then boiled in a small pan of clean water for five minutes. Many patients prefer to sterilize their syringe and needle by keeping them in a small covered dish of alcohol. Rubbing or medicated alcohol may be used, but it must be rinsed out of the syringe and needle before filling with insulin to avoid inactivation of

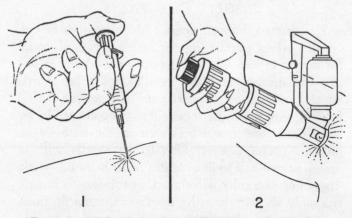

Figure 4. THE OLD AND THE NEW INJECTORS

The traditional needle and syringe (**1**) places insulin or other drugs under the skin or in a muscle. The Hypospray jet injector (**2**) does not break the skin but delivers the medication by forcing a fine spray through the skin wall.

the insulin by these types of alcohol. The ideal alcohol solution is isopropyl or ethyl alcohol of 70 per cent strength. No rinsing is necessary since this alcohol has no effect on the insulin.

Insulin need not be refrigerated except when it is being stored for more than several weeks. A week's supply can be kept in the medicine cabinet or on the dresser at room temperature. Before NPH or Lente insulin is measured out, the vial should be rolled between the palms of the hand to mix it. It should not be shaken violently lest air bubbles form which make accurate measurement difficult. Before the needle is inserted in the vial, the rubber stopper of the bottle should be wiped with alcohol-saturated cotton. The plunger is pulled back to the number of units to be withdrawn and the needle is then inserted into the vial. The barrel is pushed up and down a few times to remove air bubbles before the syringe is finally filled with insulin.

The key to painless insulin injections is speed and making sure the alcohol is dry on the needle and the syringe. After dabbing the injection area with alcohol, the diabetic should quickly insert the needle, as he would throw a dart, depressing the plunger as soon as the needle is in the skin and then withdrawing it swiftly. It is amazing how little pain there is when insulin is administered in this dart-throwing method. Slowly pushing a needle through the skin and gradually emptying the contents of the syringe can be painful. The faster the injection, the less the discomfort.

Although most diabetics grow more or less used to the needle, few individuals actually enjoy pricking their skin every day. For years, the R. P. Scherer

Corporation of Detroit has been experimenting with a needleless injector which forces the fluid painlessly through the skin by means of a jet spray. Called the Hypospray jet injector, it can use a regular vial of either U-40 or U-80 insulin. The injector works on the principle of an air rifle, and is cocked with a heavy spring.

Since the diabetic administers his own injections, the best site is the thigh. The injections can be given one inch apart in the area from the hip down to the knee, starting on the outside of the thigh, working up the middle, and then down again on the inside. Insulin injections can be rotated to include areas on the abdomen. They should not be given regularly in the arm because occasionally fatty atrophy or depressions may develop and these can be unsightly. These areas of insulin atrophy can develop in any place in the body at the site of insulin injection. The cause is unknown and there is no treatment available for it. One can prevent it by not using the same spot for the insulin injection more frequently than once a month.

INSULIN REACTIONS

Allergylike reactions to insulin occasionally develop during the first few weeks of administration, but these symptoms usually vanish after two or three weeks. These reactions consist of local itching, swelling, or pain. Naturally, the physician wants to know about these and he will treat them, generally with an antihistamine, if they persist.

Virtually every diabetic taking insulin is likely at some time to experience another form of insulin reaction. The patient's failure to follow his diet, the failure of his digestive system to dispose properly of the food he has eaten, overexertion, or too large a dose of insulin, all can produce reactions in the diabetic.

Insulin reactions will occur according to a chemical timetable determined by the type of insulin used by the patient. Reactions to regular insulin, which is rapidly absorbed into the bloodstream, usually occur three or four hours after the injection, whereas reactions to intermediate insulins can occur from eight to twenty hours after injection. That is, most patients will experience reactions between 4 P.M. and 8 P.M. It is rare for reactions to occur during the night, but occasionally too much insulin or too little blood sugar over a period of several days will cause frequent nightmares or early morning headaches—an "insulin hangover."

Some patients rarely experience insulin reactions, while others suffer them frequently. Although usually mild, insulin reactions can terrify the uninformed patient, his family, or his friends.

By understanding a little about how the body functions, especially in diabetes, the patient or his family will realize that when he is planning to exercise more vigorously than usual, a little extra carbohydrate—perhaps in the form of a soft drink—will ward off reactions. Such a precaution is especially advisable before the patient goes swimming, for an insulin reaction while he is in the water could be disastrous.

Another preventive measure is recognition of the early warning symptoms which precede an insulin reaction—increased hunger, faintness, or a cold sweat. At these signs, the alert patient should promptly drink a glass of orange juice and eat some crackers. The crackers and orange juice, which is the form of carbohydrate absorbed fastest by the body, will usually relieve the preliminary symptoms within fifteen minutes.

A patient should carry a card on his person indicating that he is a diabetic and supplying directions for treating him in an emergency. Such cards, which indicate whether the patient is taking insulin and his diet, are available from physicians. The insulin-dependent diabetic should give his friends and relatives certain basic instructions in case he goes into insulin reaction. The first rule is to ignore all the hot gossip and neighborly diagnoses for insulin reaction. Regardless of what Aunt Martha insists is the best therapy for a reaction, candy should not be used—except in an emergency when nothing else is available. This would be particularly unwise for a child who might develop an unhealthy craving for candy. Also, treating a reaction with sweets can disrupt the control of the disease.

Should the patient suffer a severe reaction, he may become delirious, or unconscious, and might not be able to swallow. Therefore, solid foods or any liquids should never be given to anyone suffering a severe reaction or unconsciousness, since they might get into the lungs and cause serious difficulties. The best treatment is to dissolve a spoonful of sugar in a little water and spoon this mixture slowly into the unconscious diabetic's mouth. Even if the patient is unconscious, he will swallow enough to relieve the reaction. If the patient is completely unconscious or is having convulsions, a physician should be called at once. If one cannot be reached, the patient's family will have to administer an emergency injection of glucagon, a substance produced by the pancreas which has the ability to elevate the blood sugar level by releasing stored sugar products from the liver. Most diabetics taking insulin are urged by their doctors to keep a supply of glucagon at home in case of emergency. A rule of thumb for the family in determining when to use glucagon is that it should be given when sugar cannot be administered by mouth. Glucagon (made by Eli Lilly & Co.) comes in a powder form with a liquid dilutant. The total amount of solution is drawn from the vial with a regular insulin syringe and injected into the vial containing the powder. The powder dissolves immediately and an insulin syringe is filled with the total amount of fluid from the ampule, and the injection is administered in the buttocks. Patients will usually respond to this injection within five to ten minutes, at which time food or orange juice can be given to prevent a recurrence of the reaction.

Occasional mild reactions need not alarm the diabetic, for they are rarely harmful. Severe reactions, with unconsciousness or convulsions, are quite serious and usually indicate gross carelessness in diet, insulin use, and exercise. They are also dangerous for others, since insulin reaction in a driver is as much a menace on the highway as alcohol. Automobile accidents involving diabetics usually occur before meals, when they are either driving to work on an empty stomach or driving home just before the evening meal. When operating a car within two hours of his next meal, the diabetic should always take some extra carbohydrate before starting off, no matter how long he has gone without insulin reactions.

POOR CONTROL AND THE DIABETIC COMA

Ketoacidosis is a complication of insulin-dependent diabetes which results when too much of the body's fat is converted to acid. When the pancreas fails to produce enough insulin to burn the sugar needed to provide fuel for physical energy, the body relies on the fat-converted-to-acid to supply these needs. The accumulation of these acid bodies in the bloodstream produces the symptoms of diabetic ketoacidosis. The appearance of ketoacidosis is often preceded by intensive thirst, rapid weight loss, and frequent urination. Principal symptoms of ketoacidosis are gastrointestinal—loss of appetite, nausea, vomiting, and abdominal pain. This last symptom is often the most severe, for the pain can resemble that of acute appendicitis or a ruptured peptic ulcer. Another sign of ketoacidosis is a hunger for air, also called "Kussmaul's breathing," which is marked by labored inhalation and exhalation. When ketoacidosis develops slowly, however, it can grow to severe proportions without any noticeable change in breathing.

Ketoacidosis sometimes appears before a patient has been diagnosed as diabetic, or in diagnosed cases in which diet and insulin requirement have been grossly neglected. In a diabetic this condition can be touched off by other factors, especially stress. Infections, major surgery, accidents, severe emotional upset, and pregnancy are stressful situations which can trigger ketoacidosis in insulin-dependent diabetes.

Early diagnosis of ketoacidosis is in the hands of the patient or his family, for any time the warning symptoms appear his urine must be tested immediately for the presence of sugar and acetone. If ketoacidosis is indeed present, sugar levels will be higher and acetone will be found. Once the preliminary diagnosis has been made, the physician will determine the most practical form of treatment. If the ketoacidosis is severe, the patient probably will require hospitalization in order to receive large amounts of insulin and fluid intravenously. However, the typical ketoacidosis is one which can be treated by increasing the insulin requirement and having the patient drink large quantities of water. At this point, close cooperation between patient and physician is essential, for one false step could lead to diabetic coma. If the patient neglects the doctor's instructions, the ketoacidosis progresses, inducing thirst, frequent urination, heavy sleepiness, and eventual unconsciousness.

There is nothing routine about diabetic coma. It is an emergency as great as or greater than the emergency of appendicitis. The patient in coma must be treated immediately if he is to live. The outcome of the coma depends on how long the patient has been unconscious before treatment is started. Until the discovery of insulin, diabetic coma marked the finale of the diabetic's short life. Today, however, coma rarely occurs, but it is a serious enough threat to encourage the prudent diabetic to be sure that friends or relatives know where he is at all times. Prolonged privacy is a luxury which the insulin diabetic cannot afford. Thus, hunting or fishing trips are permissible only when the diabetic is accompanied by a friend who knows how to treat him in case of an emergency and how to contact the patient's physician.

Ketoacidosis, like insulin reaction, should be prevented rather than treated. Infection or other forms of stress may temporarily lower the insulin requirements, and appropriate measures should be taken. Even when his stomach is upset, it is important that the diabetic always take all the daily required insulin dose, even though he may be afraid that he will be unable to eat a full meal because of continual vomiting, and thus qualify for an insulin reaction. There may be a sharp drop in food consumption during stress, but the daily insulin dose probably will not be sufficient and the diabetic will need extra insulin. The reason for this is that stress raises the blood sugar level.

Any time an insulin-dependent diabetic develops an infection or fever or starts to vomit, he should test his urine, check his body temperature, and call his doctor as soon as possible. Throughout such an illness the diabetic or a member of his family must zealously check his urine for sugar and acetone four times daily, before meals and at bedtime. Whenever the tests reveal sugar, an additional dose of rapid-acting insulin must be administered. If the stomach discomfort is so great as to prevent the patient from taking a liquid diet, he can be fed small amounts of regular ginger ale rather than the sugar-free variety.

Some individuals with sensitive stomachs develop nausea and lose their appetites during emotional upset, or when certain foods disagree with them, or during the menstrual period. If such a patient is unable to eat and yet he knows he does not have an infection, he should first check his temperature and urine. If he finds a high trace of sugar in the urine, he should take a full daily dose of insulin. If there is a slight trace of sugar, half the total daily dose should be taken as intermediate or prolonged-action insulin. The balance of the insulin dose should be taken as regular insulin in small amounts. As soon as possible he should start replacing the carbohydrates in the missed meal in the form of nondietetic ginger ale or cola, and then switching to an all-liquid diet. If vomiting persists or the patient is still unable to eat by the next meal, the physician should be contacted promptly, because inability to retain food and fluid—especially with loss of fluid from vomiting—can lead to ketoacidosis even without infection.

EXERCISE

In contrast to the invalid status assigned to diabetics before the insulin era, the diabetic today requires regular physical exercise. Because physical activity reduces blood sugar just as insulin does, exercise should be part of the daily routine. This is not much of a problem with adults, whose exercise patterns are relatively stable. Children and adolescents, however, are notoriously erratic in their daily habits, and the parents of diabetic children must vigilantly see that the patient gets about the same amount of exercise every day. Unusual or unexpected physical exertion is often quite common, but insulin-dependent diabetics can compensate for this vigorous activity either by reducing their insulin dosage or by increasing their food intake.

Many physicians and virtually all diabetics favor the latter alternative. Also, a youngster often does not know in the morning when he is giving himself his daily insulin injection that he will be participating in an impromptu football game that afternoon or that he will be invited to a beach party that evening. The extra nourishment should be taken immediately before the strenuous exercise and should consist principally of carbohydrate. When the diabetic is an active young adult who likes to play tennis or swim on weekends, he should work out every day during the week (calisthenics or other exercises) in order

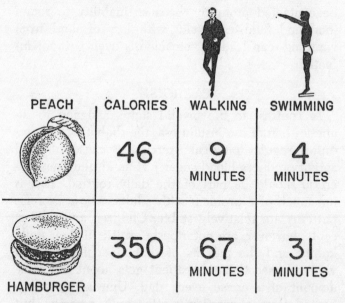

PEACH	CALORIES	WALKING	SWIMMING
	46	9 MINUTES	4 MINUTES
HAMBURGER	350	67 MINUTES	31 MINUTES

Figure 5. CALORIES AND EXERCISE

This illustrates the table in Appendix B, which gives the exercise equivalents necessary to consume the calories of typical foods.

to reduce the effect of the vigorous exercise on his disease.

Every insulin-dependent diabetic should determine his own "exercise index"—that is, the amount of extra carbohydrate needed or the number of units of insulin to be decreased for the specific kind of exercise he performs in order to prevent an insulin reaction. Only by determining his exercise index can he safely perform his needed physical activities, whether they are competitive sports or hard work. For example, a twenty-eight-year-old insulin-dependent diabetic works as a carpenter. When he is active on the job he takes thirty units of intermediate-action insulin, but on the days he loafs at home he takes forty units. Thus his exercise index is ten units of insulin for his carpentry work. All insulin-dependent diabetics should determine their own insulin and exercise needs by careful trial and error. A list of energy equivalents of food calories expressed in minutes of activity is given in Appendix B.

THE DIABETIC CHILD

Diabetes is cruelest when it strikes in childhood, for it cheats the growing youngster of one of life's most sensuous experiences—consuming pounds of candy and gallons of soft drinks. Diabetes is rough on a child, but it can be even more difficult for the child's parents—who must be masterful psychologists, skilled tacticians, and firm disciplinarians. While insisting that their youngster follow his diet and insulin schedule strictly, the parents must anticipate the many emotional and temperamental crises of childhood. This is difficult enough if there is only one child in the family, but often there are brothers and sisters whose psyches can be just as demanding as a diabetic's.

Whether a child's initial symptoms are explosive—climaxed by a diabetic coma—or mild, the diagnosis of diabetes invariably stuns the parents, especially when they are confronted with the problem of their child's survival. The initial shock gradually dissipates after the youngster is released from the hospital and the parents realize that diabetes is a permanent disease. Although fathers tend to accept this news with resignation, mothers are much more bitter and less trustful. The most difficult pill for parents to swallow is that the child has inherited the disease from one of them—even though both parents may never develop the disease. This is because diabetes is what geneticists call a *recessive* trait; that is, it is passed on through many generations but does not appear in every member of the family.

It is unfair for parents to blame themselves for a child's diabetes, for they may not have even known the disease was present in their families. Unfortunately, most parents of newly diagnosed diabetic youngsters go through a period of intense guilt, self-castigation, and mutual recrimination. It is not uncommon to find parents arguing bitterly in the waiting room of the hospital where their son or daughter is being helped through the acute phase of diabetes onset. This is particularly true when there is no clear evidence of which side of the family the disease came from. The bickering of parents determined to blame each other for carrying the disease is not likely to be conducted in discreet whispers. Thus, the child quickly learns that his diabetes

was inherited, and often he becomes resentful or
even openly enraged at his parents. Unless parents know how to counteract this rage, they and the
child will be in for some unpleasantness with an uncontrolled disease. The child's anger and resentment
can lead to calculated disobedience, a form of de-
fiance that can be frightening when the youngster
thinks he can avenge himself on his parents by not
taking his insulin or by ignoring his dietary restrictions. In such temperamental eruptions, a severe insulin reaction or even diabetic coma usually scare
even the most truculent children out of their mis-
behavior.

The diabetic child often finds it difficult to recon-
cile the capriciousness of heredity in inflicting the
disease on him and not on his brothers or sisters.
And the other children in the family can easily nour-
ish a resentment against the diabetic child when all
the parental concern and solicitude is directed toward one rather than all. In effect, the diabetic child
must receive considerable attention, yet he should
not know it. The parents can show no partiality in
matters of favors or discipline yet they must im-
press on the other children how to take care of the
afflicted one in case of trouble. The healthy children
should also be warned against using diabetes as a
weapon against the diabetic, such as by taunting him
with forbidden candy or pizza. This can be a problem with children in the early grades of school, who
tend to be more naturally mischievous and unkind
toward their brothers and sisters.

Self-Care. The faster the child is completely in-
dependent, the happier both he and his parents will
be. This is not selfishness but common sense. It is

depressing to see a fifteen-year-old leaving a urine specimen in a bottle for his mother to test or baring his leg for her to administer an insulin injection. A child so dependent on his parent is asking for trouble, and a parent who thinks it heartless to make the child take care of himself is a fool.

Surprisingly, most children are anxious to gain independence from their parents just as early as they can. A three-year-old often can start testing his urine if his parents turn the procedure into a game in which everyone guesses what color the tablet or paper strip or solution will turn. Within a few years most children are capable of performing urine tests themselves, and by nine years all children should be testing their urine without any help. The psychological benefits of this independence should not be overlooked, for the child of eight or nine tends to be concerned with personal privacy and he often resents his trips to the bathroom becoming an occasion for family togetherness.

Independence of parental help with the insulin injection comes a little later. By the time he is nine he should start giving himself injections occasionally, with a parent watching closely. The complete technique can usually be mastered by the time the youngster is ten or eleven.

Diabetics in School. Special schools are not necessary for diabetic children, but they are definitely special students, requiring the understanding and patience of the teacher. Many physicians instruct their young patients to have a midmorning snack to prevent late-morning insulin reaction. Such youngsters may become self-conscious and ashamed about this necessity around third or fourth grade—usually because eating in class makes them feel apart from the herd.

During childhood, diabetes is erratic and unstable, pouring sugar into the urine and causing frequent urination. In enlightened educational systems, in which children are permitted to leave the room quietly, this is not a major problem. In many schools, however, a medieval regimentation forces children to raise their hands and formally request permission—in front of the entire class—to visit the bathroom. Thus the diabetic child, who is already hypersensitive to his frequent need to urinate, is doubly hurt by having publicly to announce each urination. Because of the teacher's ignorance or impatience and the snickering of his fellow pupils, the very young diabetic often restrains himself and as a result wets his pants in class—an occasion for increased hilarity for the pupils and annoyance for the teacher.

The social embarrassment and humiliation usually disappear by the time the student enters the upper grades and high school. The problem then becomes one of scheduling, for the diabetic youngster requires a special schedule to avoid insulin reactions. For example, physical education classes should be taken after lunch instead of immediately before. Occasionally the diabetic pupil who has a midmorning gym class will do poorly in the class immediately following it because of an unrecognized insulin reaction.

Educational ignorance is a serious nuisance which can complicate the life of the diabetic unnecessarily. Many teachers with afflicted students have made an effort to learn about the disease and how to handle it, but others are still shamefully ignorant. The uninformed teachers often regard insulin reactions and frequent urination as behavior problems, and as affronts to their authority. This can lead to open warfare between teacher and pupil, with the teacher needling, nagging, and harassing the child for every error. In such cases a phone call from the physician to the principal or the teacher often resolves the conflict.

More common is the "little bit of knowledge" syndrome, especially popular among physical education instructors. Having once heard that exercise can sometimes be dangerous for diabetics, the instructors forbid even the most ordinary routines and prevent diabetics from joining any teams. Usually the youngster's physician can avoid such situations by certifying that the diabetic may participate in any sports he wishes as long as he takes extra carbohydrate (a sugared soft drink or a glass of orange juice) before indulging.

Note to Teachers: The primary problem with diabetic pupils is insulin reaction, recognizing it immediately, and counteracting it. In elementary school children reactions usually occur just before noon or around 3 P.M., the times when the insulin reaches its peak action. These reactions can be traced to excess exercise, too much insulin, decreased food intake, or irregular living habits (also known as "hypertelevisionosis," a condition marked by sleepiness and eyestrain).

When a teacher discovers that she has an insulin-dependent diabetic in her class, it is wise to confer immediately with the parents. Occasionally a chat with the child's physician and the school nurse is helpful in anticipating difficulties and learning how to handle any emergencies. School nurses will usually put in a supply of glucagon in case the reaction is so severe that orange juice or other carbohydrates cannot be swallowed.

Like parents, teachers must be constantly vigilant but not overly solicitous or protective. There is no reason the child cannot participate normally in school activities, provided diet and insulin dosage are regulated according to the amount of exercise taken each day. The teacher who knows her pupil's condition and how to treat any emergencies can then pretend not to notice the youngster or show him any extra attention. This will permit the child to be absorbed into the class, and will help prevent future emotional problems.

Camps for Diabetic Children. The idea of whisking diabetic children off to special camps each summer has gained popularity in the last thirty years —perhaps because both children and parents need and enjoy a vacation from each other. For the youngster it's a splendid chance to spring free from parental supervision and romp around outdoors, participate in sports, and generally let off steam in a well-protected environment of fellow diabetics and trained personnel. Camp is an ideal place for the overly dependent child to learn complete self-reliance from those who have already mastered it. He learns how to test his own urine, and obtains some knowledge about diet and food. Under the observation of trained counselors, the physicians and nurses of the staff, he gets his diet, exercise, and insulin in the right proportions.

One disadvantage of diabetic camps is the psychological impact of throwing the docile, naïve child together with a strong-willed child who is beginning to rebel against his parents, his doctor, the camp authorities, or even against his disease and the precautions necessary to keep it in control. The danger is that the naïve child may be attracted to the stronger personality of the rebel and seek to imitate him. If the older youngster is in apparent good health and also spreading his doctrine of resistance and revolution, the younger child may logically conclude that diet, daily insulin injections, and regular testing of the urine are insidious devices of parents and doctors to keep him under their collective thumb. This line of reasoning sounds silly to a mature adult, but it is precisely the way a previously docile, well-behaved child will first react to the seeds of rebellion. When such a child returns home from camp, preaching sedition and overthrow of parental authority, the indignant parents are likely to assume that little Oscar would not have become this way except for the evil influences of diabetic camp. This is not really true, however, for almost all children rebel at some time, in some manner, and it might even be better to expose a child to this possibility at camp in order to get it out of his system before the agonies of adolescence strike.

Another minor drawback to the camp that admits both boys and girls is the possibility that two diabetics might form a friendship that could lead ultimately to marriage and the probability of passing the disease on to children. This possibility is thwarted both by the camp's refusal to accept youngsters older than sixteen and by the diabetics themselves, who are well aware of the hereditary nature of their disease.

There are over fifty diabetic camps in the United States, scattered throughout the country. A list of these camps can be obtained from the American Diabetes Association, 18 E. 48th Street, New York 10017, N. Y.

Adolescent Diabetics. The combination of a serious disease with the emotional and physical uproar of the teens is frightening in its potential, yet somehow both teen-agers and their parents survive. During these years, however, the wise parent realizes that the disease is likely to slip out of control from time to time, but an attitude of detached watchfulness and patient understanding will keep domestic life relatively tranquil. Naturally, there will be crises, but the parent should take them in stride, with as little emotional involvement as possible. It is always hard for parents to keep their noses out of their children's lives, but it is especially difficult during adolescence when youngsters seem intent on doing everything possible to infuriate their parents.

Trouble can come from almost any direction to a teen-age diabetic, even when the youngster is behaving rationally, following his diet, and taking insulin regularly. It can result from a sudden burst of intensive physical activity or from emotional tensions over a difficult exam or a red-hot love affair.

Rebellion against the disciplines of diabetes management is common but transient. The daily routine of insulin, urine testing, diet, and exercise can be sufficiently tedious to tempt the young diabetic to grow careless and indifferent. The worst antidote to this is parental sternness, dramatically accompanied by threats and intimidation. Any punitive or restrictive action will only worsen the situation. The moody melodrama of adolescence passes quickly if ignored, but can become dangerous when nourished by needling or nagging. This often leads to self-pity, which induces the diabetic to try to punish his parents or his girl friend or his teachers by letting his disease get out of control. This is usually a subconscious desire, but occasionally the punishment urge becomes explicit in a drive toward self-destruction.

An extreme example of this was an eighteen-year-old boy who stomped up to his room and banged the door shut after a violent quarrel with his mother. Tears streaming down his face, he loaded his syringe with regular insulin and gave himself what he was sure would be a lethal injection. When his mother called upstairs to ask if he had cooled off, the boy shouted, "You'll be sorry for what you've done to me! And you'll never have a chance to apologize!" Somewhat alarmed, his mother hurried to his room, where she found the empty insulin ampule and syringe. The boy was sobbing into his pillow, denouncing her and the rest of the world for not understanding him, etc. She called the doctor, asking if she should rush the boy to the hospital. "That really won't be necessary," he assured her, instructing her instead to prepare for a hair-raising insulin reaction which would be unpleasant for the boy but would not kill him. The physician advised her to give him several glasses of orange juice and, if he became unconscious, to give him an injection of glucagon. If after one hour he still had not recovered, he should be seen by the doctor.

This is an extreme, of course, but most parents of adolescent diabetics experience similar unpleasant crises. The wisest way to handle these and avoid repeat performances is to be moderate in all aspects of parenthood, avoiding overprotectiveness, resentment, annoyance with the disease's inconvenience to the rest of the family, and coddling. It is difficult to be more specific than this, for no two teen-agers are alike and their problems vary in degree and intensity too extensively for generalization.

Not all adolescent problems are emotional or psychological. At some point during the teen years, bodily growth causes a burst of appetite which in turn must be countered by increased insulin dosage. Another nutritional headache is the tendency of a teen-ager to gallop along with the herd as it moves from hot-dog stand to pizzeria. It is easy to preach firmness of character and moral restraint, but few adolescents are willing to incur the contempt of the mob—even if it means wolfing down thousands of extra calories.

Social conformity also intrudes on the teen-age diabetic at parties, picnics, and beach outings. Few adolescents think twice about hopping into a swimsuit and splashing in the surf, but diabetics are often hypersensitive if there are needle marks on their thighs. Another socially awkward problem is whether a diabetic should tell the opposite sex that he has diabetes. As dating partnerships get more involved, reticence usually disappears and he tells his friends about his disease.

Various local diabetes associations have organized

vocational and counseling services to help not only the adult diabetic with problems of vocation, family, insurance, and other problems, but also the young person whose problems are complicated by diabetes. The teen-ager and young adult are invited to participate in group discussion sessions, run by a consulting psychologist, social worker, and physician. In these, over a period of five to six months, they explore areas of vocational selection, education, family life, social life, marriage, and many other aspects of living which may involve the presence of diabetes.

Career Planning. Certain careers are not open to diabetics. Diabetic boys are barred from joining the police and from firefighting, military service, commercial piloting, or any other conveying of passengers. Girls cannot become airline stewardesses and are often prevented from teaching or nursing. The principal reason for these closed doors is the possibility of an insulin reaction at a dangerous moment. A secondary reason is simple job discrimination, which prevents diabetics from being hired for non-dangerous jobs (such as teaching) on the grounds that they would miss too many working days. This, of course, is poppycock, for diabetic workers whose disease is under control have a lower absentee rate than their healthy brethren. Many industrial firms have an irrevocable policy against hiring diabetics, and should a long-term employee suddenly develop the disease, out he goes. And the New York City Board of Education—whose school system is among the nation's worst—also discriminates against diabetic teachers. Fortunately, some of the ignorance of job discrimination has been battered down by the diabetes associations, but there is still much more that has to be done. Evangelical work can be performed by successfully employed insulin-dependent diabetics who, by careful management of their disease, have avoided insulin reactions or ketoacidosis on the job.

CHAPTER 7

Type B:
Overweight Diabetes

Overweight diabetes is the most common and, until recently, the least understood form of the disease. More than 80 per cent of all cases fall into the Type B classification, which is also known as maturity-onset or stable adult diabetes. It generally appears after forty years of age, and its victims are almost always overweight. The key to successful treatment of overweight diabetes is that insulin should not be used, lest the patient's weight increase and thus worsen the disease.

Diabetes develops in the obese patient very slowly and is quite insidious in its onset. This can be seen in the case of Ruth K. a fifty-year-old housewife who had been overweight for many years. Her father and two of her sisters had diabetes. She noticed that recently she was getting quite tired and dizzy. She did not notice any increase in her thirst or appetite, but because of her family history of diabetes, she consulted her doctor. He did blood- and urine-sugar tests two hours after she had eaten a typical high-carbohydrate breakfast of a large glass of orange juice, two slices of toast with jelly, eggs, and coffee with sugar. Her blood sugar level was over 250 milligrams and there was a large amount of sugar in her urine but no acetone. Her physician told her that her first concern should be to lose at least twenty-five pounds. He put her on a 1000-calorie diet and prescribed an oral hypoglycemic agent,

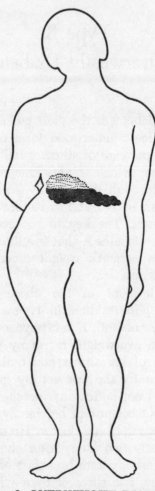

Figure 6. OVERWEIGHT DIABETES

The insulin production is adequate, but part of it (speckled area) is inactive. This type of diabetes is the most common of all and usually doesn't strike until middle age. Its favorite victims are overweight women.

and she learned how to test her urine for sugar and, when necessary, acetone. The following week her physician performed an exhaustive physical examination, including an electrocardiogram, chest X ray, blood count, and urinalysis. He found her blood pressure had increased and he prescribed a low-salt diet, avoiding highly salted foods such as peanuts, ham, bacon, etc. He also gave her a prescription for a drug to reduce the blood pressure. After three months she had lost twenty-two pounds, her urine was almost sugar-free, and her blood pressure had returned to normal. Her dizziness and fatigue had disappeared, and she felt better than she had in a long time.

Overweight diabetes acts very differently from insulin-dependent diabetes. Type B victims might have high blood sugar levels, but they are not likely to develop ketoacidosis. In 1955, investigators first noted that these diabetics, when administered insulin, increased their weight and blood sugar levels in direct proportion to any rise in their insulin dosage. When the insulin was decreased, however, the blood sugar levels dropped, as did the weight. In an occasional case the overweight diabetics could be gradually reduced from eighty units of insulin per day to ten, then five, and finally none at all. And the blood sugar levels remained lower without the insulin than they had been while insulin was regularly injected.

THE DEVELOPMENT OF ORAL DRUGS

The basic physiological explanation of this phenomenon was provided by the development of the oral hypoglycemic drugs. Although the principle was first discovered in 1942, the war interfered with any additional investigation. They were studied during the late 1940s and early 1950s in Germany, resulting in the introduction of carbutamide or BZ-55 in 1954 in Germany. Although it is still used in Europe, carbutamide has never won much of a fan club in the United States, for when it was studied here it was found to produce a number of dangerous side reactions affecting the blood, bone marrow, and liver.

In 1956 the first oral hypoglycemic drug, tolbutamide, was introduced in the United States by the Upjohn Company. Marketed under the brand name of *Orinase,* tolbutamide was found to lower blood sugar levels without causing the side effects or toxic reactions of carbutamide. Tolbutamide, which belongs to a group of drugs known as the sulfonylureas, was followed by two similar compounds, chlorpropamide (*Diabinese,* Charles Pfizer & Co.) and acetohexamide (*Dymelor,* Eli Lilly & Co.). These sulfonylureas stimulate the cells of the pancreas to release insulin, which in turn lowers blood sugar levels.

Phenformin, a completely different type of drug belonging to the chemical family called the biguanides, was developed and then introduced in 1959 under the trade name of *DBI* by the U.S. Vitamin Corp. Unlike the sulfonylureas, phenformin does not depend on the functioning beta cells of the pancreas to reduce excess blood sugar. Instead, phenformin's action appears to stimulate intracellular glycolysis, a chemical process by which the sugar or glucose is broken down into more readily usable fuel for the cells. It acts by burning up sugar in the muscles and other tissues. It does not stimulate the pancreas to produce more insulin, as do the sulfonylureas.

The use of oral drugs gained immediate popularity, but physicians were uncertain for several years what their over-all effect would be in the long-term treatment of overweight diabetes. Detailed studies of the basic physiology of diabetes soon began to throw light on the hitherto uncharted aspects of the disease.

Measurements of insulin activity in the overweight diabetic revealed that such patients often had a normal amount of insulin present in the bloodstream. This was especially true when the insulin circulating in the blood was measured immediately after a high-carbohydrate meal. This meant that the carbohydrate stimulated insulin production. However, not all of this insulin was being effectively used by the diabetic's system, and some of it appeared to be inactive and incapable of burning up all the carbohydrate dumped into the bloodstream by the diet. This supply of partially incompetent insulin is the reason such individuals are diabetic and, because there is no insulin deficiency they are not insulin-dependent.

THE ROLE OF EXCESS WEIGHT

Another paradox of Type B diabetes is the important role played by excess weight. The overweight diabetic who successfully peels off enough pounds to get his weight back to normal usually experiences a dramatic improvement in his condition. Indeed, the symptoms often virtually disappear. Weight reduction and control can bring this incurable disease closer to complete remission than any medication. This is because excess weight usually creates an increased demand for insulin by the body. The more body fat, the more insulin is required. Insulin is the body's most potent fat-producing hormone and it stimulates the appetite. If this vicious cycle is broken, the patient's insulin needs drop to normal levels.

Why then are there any diabetics of the overweight type, if weight reduction accomplishes so much? The answer is rooted, not in the pancreas or the liver, but rather in the psyche. Very few individuals—diabetic or not—can or will follow a strict diet long enough to get their weight down and keep it at normal levels.

Even when the diabetic is willing and cooperative, it is not easy to lose weight. There are some medical crutches which sometimes are helpful. Pills which suppress the appetite (amphetamines, etc.) can be prescribed, but the patient must be able to tolerate their stimulating action. Other methods that occasionally succeed are psychotherapy or group obesity clinics.

When weight loss is crucial, the sulfonylureas, which stimulate insulin, should not be used. Phenformin, on the other hand, is more effective in treating obese diabetics, for it does not cause the pancreas to produce more insulin and stimulate weight increase. Before phenformin was developed, the obese patient who took any of the sulfonylureas continued to gain weight. The more weight gained, the worse the diabetes became. However, after a period of taking phenformin and dieting to reduce their body weight, their condition generally improved.

CHAPTER 8

Type AB:
Stress Diabetes

Stress diabetes is the newest form of diabetes. That is, Type AB has only recently been recognized and classified. It is called stress diabetes because the patients normally can be controlled with oral drugs or small doses of insulin, but physical or emotional stress will sharply increase their blood sugar. Stress diabetes first appears in men and women in their thirties or forties who are either underweight or of normal weight. The disease responds well to oral hypoglycemic therapy, and if it is diagnosed while still mild, the disease usually shows most of the symptoms of overweight diabetes—except that the victims are not overweight.

During times of stress—infections, surgery, or emotional crises—the Type AB patient often must be transferred from oral therapy to insulin injections, or if they are already on insulin, their insulin requirements increase. Occasionally, prolonged stress will turn an AB stress diabetic into a Type A insulin-dependent diabetic, one who develops a true insulin deficiency and needs insulin the rest of his life.

An interesting illustration of stress diabetes is the case of Paul S., a thirty-nine-year-old advertising account executive in New York. He was the very model of the well-adjusted, socially popular ad man, with a wife and two children living in a ranch house in a Westchester suburb. He rode the same train to work every day, played bridge with the same gang, and always held stylishly correct, noncontroversial opinions on all popular topics. In short, Paul was a healthy, well-rounded, typical American, but rather dull. His life threatened to continue on its humdrum course until an unexpected merger of his agency with a larger firm left Paul without a job. For two days he worried about how he would keep up with the mortgage, car, and washing machine payments. Then an old friend at another agency called him at home and told Paul he could have a better job at a higher salary.

For several days after he had lost his job, Paul felt fatigued and thirstier than usual. His wife suggested that he see a doctor for a checkup, but Paul pointed out that he had always been in excellent health. He did, however, agree to see his family physician, who found sugar in Paul's urine as well as an elevated blood sugar level.

Since he was not truly insulin-dependent, the doctor said Paul was not Type A, but he certainly lacked some of the prime characteristics of Type B. Therefore, his diabetes was probably the uncertain Type AB, or stress diabetes. Paul would have to be watched closely over a long period of time, and he would have to keep accurate records of his emotional and physical ups and downs. Although his diabetes seemed the mildest of the three types, it was also the least trustworthy—its behavior was completely undependable.

Paul returned immediately to his regular pattern of commuting, bridge playing, golf every weekend, two martinis before supper, and lots of television each night. Far from being self-conscious or embarrassed about his diabetes, Paul crowed to his commuting colleagues about his rare type of disease. It was certainly a more interesting condition than the standard suburban ulcer.

Paul had all but forgotten about his disease two years later when one day he answered his phone at the office and was told that his twelve-year-old daughter had been run over by a taxi. The girl was in critical condition with multiple fractures and a brain concussion. His wife was hysterical and had to be put under sedation.

By the time he left the hospital late that evening, his daughter was out of danger, his wife had recovered, but Paul was grimly ill. At first he thought the weakness and waves of nausea might be a normal reaction to what had just happened, but when he felt worse the next day, he called his doctor. A rapid analysis of Paul's physical condition indicated that the emotional catastrophe had triggered a change in his diabetes to temporary insulin dependence which could not be controlled by oral drugs because he had a small amount of acetone in his urine. His doctor prescribed fifteen units of insulin daily until the blood sugar levels returned to their prestress levels. This lasted for three months, and then Paul was able to resume taking the oral hypoglycemic agents.

Little is known about stress diabetes other than how it manifests itself. It can be potentially dangerous, for unless carefully followed, it can suddenly spring out of control. Stress diabetes is a "sometime thing." It is cyclical and can appear and disappear. Occasionally this type of diabetes may "mutate" or change its characteristic to insulin-dependent diabetes, requiring substantial amounts of insulin to maintain good control. This can be predicted by careful attention to the urine tests, and if acetone is present, insulin should be taken immediately.

PART IV

Living with
Diabetes

CHAPTER 9

Special Problems of Diabetics

COMPLICATIONS OF DIABETES

Poorly controlled diabetes often results in complications of the skin, nervous system, and blood vessels.

Skin: High blood sugar levels can influence the skin, producing generalized itchiness all over the body. In fact, nonstop itching is one of the most common complaints of patients with uncontrolled diabetes. The diabetic's skin is also more susceptible to infection, boils, carbuncles, abscesses, and fungus infections (such as athlete's foot). Women often experience an embarrassingly severe itch around the vulva which, when scratched vigorously, can develop into a rash with little pockets of pus. Women are also more likely than men to develop *necrobiosis lipoidica,* a skin rash which consists of oval, firm, yellowish cracks on the legs and arms. There is no specific treatment for this except frequent washing with medicated soap.

Nervous system: Diabetic neuritis is seen most frequently in the old, the obese, and those patients who spill large quantities of sugar into their urine. The first symptoms of this complication are peculiar sensations in the hands and feet, changing to alternating numbness and tingling with occasional pain. This form of neuritis is treated with large doses of vitamin B or vitamin B_{12} and by bringing the diabetes under better control. Diabetic neuropathy

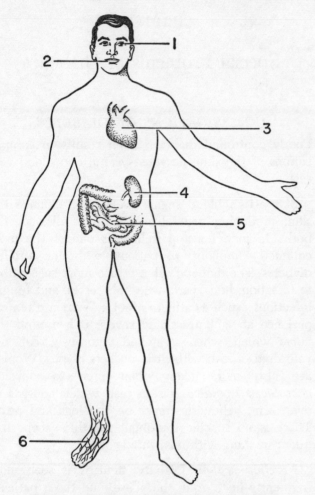

Figure 7. COMPLICATIONS OF DIABETES

The most frequent complications of diabetes affect the blood vessels in the eyes (**1**) and the blood supply to the gums, triggering assorted dental problems (**2**). Heart disease (**3**) and kidney disease (**4**) can also result from diabetes, along with gastrointestinal disorders (**5**) such as diarrhea, cramps, or spasms, and diminished circulation (**6**) throughout the body but especially in the feet.

shows up as muscle weakness of the eye or bladder, constipation, or nocturnal diarrhea. This complication is also treated with vitamins and better control of the diabetes.

Blood vessels: Retinopathy (or retinitis, as it is also known) is a potential threat to all diabetics, particularly the Type A or insulin-dependent. In this complication the blood vessels in the inner lining of the eyeball, or retina, multiply. The tiny new vessels serve no important function, but they often burst and cause little hemorrhages on the retina. These in turn result in blind spots. This condition often fluctuates in its seriousness, but ultimately the hemorrhages increase and vision diminishes. There are many forms of treatment for retinopathy, but no universally effective method has been found. Hormone therapy to inhibit the pituitary—the gland responsible for the growth of new vessels—is sometimes effective, as is implanting radioactive material in the pituitary or removing part of the gland surgically (hypophysectomy). The causes of retinopathy are still unknown. However, the condition is often found in diabetics whose disease has not always been under good control.

Occasionally diabetics develop kidney disease as a complication of diabetes. Little is known about the precise connection between the two diseases, or how the one stimulates the other. Any kidney disorder is always serious, and such a complication of diabetes will require close medical attention. Good nutrition and vitamins are the only specific therapeutics yet available.

CARE OF THE FEET

Overweight diabetes is often accompanied by foot disorders, especially among those patients over forty. The longer a person has had diabetes, the greater are his chances that his arteries will narrow and thus decrease the supply of blood to the feet. This decrease in circulation lowers resistance to infection and also reduces pain and temperature sen-

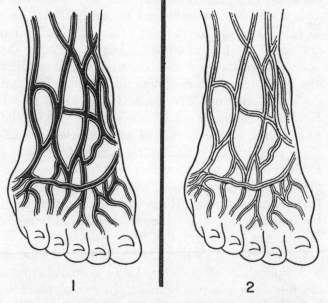

1   2

Figure 8. BLOOD CIRCULATION IN THE FEET

A normal person's blood supply to his feet (**1**) keeps the tissues adequately supplied with oxygen. A typical complication of diabetes, however, is the gradual narrowing of the arteries (**2**) until the blood flow barely trickles through. This makes any bruise, cut, or scrape a serious health menace because impaired circulation retards healing.

sation. A diabetic who has had the disease only a short time may also develop foot problems if his diabetes is out of control.

The loss of nerve sensation is dangerous because a person might pay insufficient attention to cuts, bruises, corns, or calluses, which can, if unattended, develop into serious infections. Insensitivity to excess heat can lead to severe burns, often from hot water bottles or electric heating pads. Burns or infection, when accompanied by inadequate circulation, can result in gangrene, a condition in which the tissue dies and the skin turns blue or black.

Keeping the diabetes under control increases the body's resistance to infection, diminishes the likelihood of gangrene, and prevents the arteries from narrowing. Another preventive measure is to keep the skin intact. Any cracks or breaks (as a result of cuts, athlete's foot, ingrown toenails, poorly fitting shoes) offer bacteria an opportunity to enter the body and start infections.

There are a few handy rules for daily care of the feet:

► Wear clean socks every day.

► Soak the feet daily in warm water. Since a diabetic's feet are often not sufficiently sensitive to heat, the water temperature should be tested by dipping the elbows or wrists in first. This prevents scalds from water that is too hot.

► Clean toenails carefully with orangewood sticks.

► Cut toenails straight across to prevent the corners from catching under the skin as they grow out. Ingrown toenails can easily lead to infection.

► Shoes should be properly fitted and comfortable, preferably made with soft leather with a smooth lining. New shoes must be broken in slowly and with great care. Wear them only a few hours each day at first.

► Inspect the feet critically each day, checking for cracks, calluses, blisters, or bruises. Examine the shoes to make sure there are no rough spots in the lining. Wrap overlapping or hammer toes with lamb's wool to reduce the pressure on them.

► Never wear band-type garters that encircle the leg with elastic, either above or below the knee. Nylon stockings with built-in elastic tops are also dangerous for diabetics.

FOOT AILMENTS

Cold feet can indicate a number of complaints other than poor circulation. Nervousness and neuritis are two common causes of cold feet. When a diabetic is conscious of a distinct chilliness in his lowest extremities he may find warmth from wearing wool socks as often as possible. If the feet are cold only at night, socks worn to bed can be supplemented with an electric blanket.

Dry skin should not be peeled or scraped off, lest the skin be torn. Rather, the feet should be soaked daily, then rubbed with lanolin, olive oil, or an oil-producing skin ointment. Persistent dry skin can sometimes be overcome by changing the type of stocking material or even the shoe style.

Athlete's foot is a fungus which appears between the toes or on the soles of the feet. It frequently cracks the skin and sets off secondary infections. Although nondiabetics can treat athlete's foot themselves, the diabetic should consult his physician before he uses any of the popular cures for athlete's foot, since some of them may cause a temporary increase in inflammation. The usual therapy for a diabetic's athlete's foot is a fungicide ointment or lotion applied after the evening bath and a fungicide powder sprinkled between the toes in the morning.

Corns and calluses should never be cut, nor should local remedies be used, since they may be too harsh or harmful to the skin. Most solutions used to dissolve corns and calluses contain acid, which can cause secondary infection in the sensitive diabetic skin. Corns often can be improved by changing shoes, and calluses can be rubbed with gauze or an emery board after the foot bath to get rid of dried skin.

Cuts and bruises should be washed with soap and water, then held under tepid running water for at least one minute. Apply an antiseptic and cover with a sterile dressing. If the bandage sticks to the wound, apply a bland ointment such as vaseline or boric acid to the dressing pad. Avoid harsh antiseptics such as iodine, for those strong enough to kill bacteria are also strong enough to damage sensitive tissue. Some patients feel secure only when applying some medication, and if this is the case, tincture of merthiolate is permitted for superficial scratches. However, soap, water, and a sterile bandage are just as effective.

The worst aggravation for a swollen or infected foot is walking. Any infections, cuts, bruises, or skin breaks in a diabetic's feet should be reported to the doctor.

PREGNANCY

One of the most persistent misunderstandings about diabetes is the belief that it is almost impossible for a diabetic woman to get pregnant, and that if she does so, the baby will certainly be born dead. Although there is no truth to this legend, few could have disputed it two generations ago. The truth is that diabetes itself is not the culprit in pregnancy, but rather the physical consequences of poorly controlled diabetes.

A well-controlled diabetic woman is as fertile as a healthy woman, and the effects of pregnancy on her disease are nullified by adequate insulin therapy and by better understanding and management of toxemia, a condition which pumps poisons into the bloodstream.

But the single most important guarantee of a healthy pregnancy for both mother and child is a four-way cooperative alliance of the patient, the obstetrician, the internist* or family doctor, and the pediatrician. To ignore medical advice is considerably more dangerous for the diabetic during pregnancy. It is essential that she be seen by both her obstetrician and her internist at regular intervals throughout the pregnancy. Constant supervision by

* An internist should not be confused with an intern, a graduate medical student who serves an apprenticeship in a hospital. An internist is a physician who has completed his internship and has studied for several years more to become a specialist in internal medicine and organ systems. He is a diagnostician, consultant, and personal medical advisor. The internist, along with the general practitioner, sees and treats most cases of diabetes. Pediatricians, who specialize in the care of children, and gynecologists, specialists in women's diseases, also treat diabetes.

these two specialists will enable them to prevent serious deviations in the diabetic and quickly detect and treat those minor ones which occur.

Since diabetic acidosis is a frequent cause of miscarriages, the pregnant patient should test her urine for sugar and acetone four times daily. Her diet will have to be adjusted to keep her weight at the optimum level throughout pregnancy, and salts will probably be eliminated from her diet, especially if she has a tendency to retain fluids. The insulin dose (since virtually all pregnant women have insulin-dependent diabetes) may have to be adjusted periodically during pregnancy to ward off insulin reactions, and she may require a diuretic—a drug which gets rid of excess fluids in the body tissues.

Nausea. Morning sickness, an occasional manifestation during the first three months of pregnancy, may prove troublesome for diabetics, especially if it restricts their regular consumption of food. They can be treated with frequent doses of regular (quick-acting) insulin until the nausea has subsided and they are able to resume their normal diets. However, excessive vomiting which leads to acidosis is so serious that if it does not subside immediately, the patient may have to be hospitalized temporarily. Insulin maintenance throughout pregnancy is important in almost all diabetics, for oral hypoglycemic agents are incapable of controlling the diabetes adequately during this crucial period.

Delivery. Caesarian section used to be the standard method of delivery for diabetic mothers, but many physicians today permit the pregnancies to terminate naturally. After the obstetrician has calculated her estimated delivery date, the mother will probably enter the hospital several days early so that her diabetes can be kept under strict control throughout labor, delivery, and recuperation. If Caesarian section is to be done, it usually is performed during the thirty-sixth week of the pregnancy. Often a mother's insulin requirements will drop sharply immediately after delivery, especially during the first twenty-four hours. This is because certain anti-insulin factors are often contained in the placenta, which is shed as the "afterbirth," and also because of other hormonal controls.

The determining factor in prescribing Caesarian or normal delivery for a diabetic mother who is physiologically capable of delivering normally is the possibility of toxemia as well as how long the mother has had diabetes. Physicians generally discourage their patients from having more than three children by Caesarian section, because of the stress this places on the mother. If a diabetic mother is able to have children normally, there is no limit to the number of children she can have. However, because diabetes is an hereditary disease, most diabetic mothers choose to keep their families small.

Care of the baby. The pediatrician is usually present at birth in order to take over care of the infant. Although babies of diabetic women are often overweight (they may weigh nine to eleven pounds), all such infants are treated as prematures because their physiological development rarely corresponds to their size. They have more fat, their tissues retain more fluid, and some organs, especially the liver, are larger than normal. Sometimes they may even have jaundice at birth. Their marked loss of weight after delivery is due to the loss of the excess fluid in the tissues. The infant stays in the hospital a little longer than other babies for observation and prevention of complications.

One of the first things the pediatrician will look for is any sign of hyaline membrane disease, a respiratory complaint resembling bronchitis in which the baby has difficulty breathing properly. Although once inevitably fatal, the prognosis of hyaline membrane disease has improved considerably in recent years. Prompt recognition of the ailment and intensive care in the hospital seem to be the keys to successful management. For some reason, hyaline membrane disease has increased in children born to diabetic mothers, which is the reason why physicians examine such children thoroughly immediately after birth.

EMOTIONAL PROBLEMS

Although the emotional and psychological needs of the young diabetic are frequently discussed, not enough attention is paid to the psyche of the adult diabetic. Fear of the disease, if unrecognized by the physician, can make even the best-controlled diabetic's life hell. Even when the doctor assures the patient that there's nothing to worry about, the patient may regard this advice as 95 per cent platitude.

It is common for adult diabetics to worry excessively about deformity, blindness, incapacity, and death. Many of them pick up every available book on the topic and skim through the listings of complications to see if any new ones have been added recently. If the diabetic is too frightened to talk, or his physician too busy to carefully probe each fear and provide sound information, it might be the time to see a psychiatrist. Often a psychiatrist can get to the root of a diabetic's fears and enable him to live in emotional comfort with the disease.

A prelude to outright fear is anxiety. This often means worrying excessively about possible complications of the disease. In at least one type of situation anxiety can sometimes trigger a problem that often has been blamed on diabetes—impotence. For many years it was thought that the diminished circulation caused by diabetes had something to do with preventing diabetic men from satisfactorily performing the sex act. Physicians and psychiatrists today, however, suspect that most impotence—in diabetics and nondiabetics—is psychological rather than organic in origin. And in diabetics, anxiety is usually the cause. This is another problem area in which psychiatric assistance sometimes can be very beneficial to the diabetic.

Some patients find themselves overly dependent on their physician for control of their disease. This is not wise, for such patients become desperate with fear when the doctor is out of town or otherwise unavailable when they need him. These individuals have failed to understand properly the role of the patient in controlling diabetes, or else they cling to the doctor for psychiatric reasons.

Diabetics who find themselves depressed need not be concerned that this is a permanent part of their disease. Should it become troublesome, however, their physicians can usually treat depression easily with one of the antidepressant drugs.

EMPLOYMENT

Job discrimination against diabetics is not uncommon in the United States, and it is as absurd as the racial and ethnic discrimination which still prevails. This problem has been discussed in the section on Career Planning under Type A, insulin-dependent diabetes, since these diabetics frequently encounter prejudice and ignorance among employers. However, all diabetics are potential victims of discrimination because of their disease.

Some arguments advanced by employers for not hiring diabetics include insulin shock, prolonged absenteeism, increased compensation and more importantly, insurance costs, and the various complications of diabetes. Yet each of these objections can be overruled by good medical care, careful control of the disease, periodic examination, and intelligent job placement. A diabetic job applicant should be evaluated by the same criteria as the nondiabetic applicant. The employer, however, does have a right to know the severity of an individual's disease, how it is regulated and controlled, and if he is willing to submit to periodic examination.

The severity of the diabetes is perhaps the most important consideration in determining a man's job potential. The mildly afflicted diabetic who is controlled by diet alone or by diet and one of the oral drugs presents little problem. The insulin-dependent diabetic, however, obviously should not be responsible for transporting people or operating dangerous machinery. All diabetics should be placed in jobs in which there is no danger of injuring their lower extremities. Foot and toe accidents can easily lead to ulceration, infection, or gangrene, which in turn keep the employee out of work for long periods of time.

Occasionally a physician will turn thumbs down on an industrial job candidate who requires insulin but is poorly controlled and uncooperative. A reckless, don't-give-a-damn attitude toward insulin-dependent diabetes may signify the soul of a free spirit, but it also indicates a poor employment risk. Such a person cannot be employed in any position in which he is likely to suffer a serious accident or cause one for fellow workers. Any injury to this diabetic will probably touch off a complication, keeping him away from the job much longer than usual. The only careers suitable for such diabetics are non-dangerous, sedentary ones such as law, journalism, administration, or Holy Orders. A truculent diabetic is unfit to drive a bus, operate a bulldozer, perform on the trapeze, or serve as a lifeguard at a crowded swimming pool. However, he may be eminently capable of composing a symphony, writing indignant editorials, arguing the nuances of law or theology, or dictating prizewinning memos in virtually any executive position.

The insulin-dependent diabetic should request a regular schedule, avoiding if possible the "graveyard shift"—that is, the midnight-to-8 A.M. hours, since it is more difficult to follow a regular routine on the night shift in regard to timing of diet, exercise, disturbance in sleep during the day, and other abnormal factors.

INSURANCE

Insurance companies are not charitable organizations, and asking them to offer life or health insurance to diabetics was, until recently, usually greeted with a polite smile. Today, however, both kinds of insurance are available to diabetics, provided they maintain good control of their disease and pay higher premiums. This is a very recent development, and diabetics can assume that even the rates will drop a bit as research improves methods of treatment and control and the companies themselves learn more about underwriting chronic-disease risks. A diabetic now can obtain one of many life insurance policies provided he meet certain minimum standards and comply with various requirements. As far as insurance is concerned there is one keynote rule for diabetics: Get all you can while you can, as cheaply as you can. You may not be able to do it later.

Health insurance, however, is another matter, for each diabetic will need certain types of coverage which may not be uniformly available in all health insurance plans. No insurance company has yet offered a plan of total protection. However, by shopping intelligently, the diabetic can select an insurance that provides the kind of coverage he wants. If the patient knows an insurance agent, he should by all means consult him, along with his own physician. Naturally, any insurance contract should be carefully scrutinized to make sure all the salesman's promises are included.

What is the ideal health insurance for a diabetic? A good plan will provide for hospital care by covering at least 75 per cent of the daily room rate. The shrewd patient might first obtain the room rates of his local hospital so he can compare them with the benefits of the various policies.

But room rates are only a small part of hospital costs—especially for a diabetic. The ideal health insurance will provide generously for extra services, such as blood transfusions, intravenous medication, oxygen, antibiotics for infections, etc.

And since diabetes produces complications which must be treated, a sound health insurance plan should cover the costs of diagnostic tests (such as X rays, blood tests, laboratory analyses, catheterization, or biopsies). Insurance should cover diagnostic procedures whether they are done in the hospital or in the physician's office.

Many hospital admissions today are for nonsurgical conditions—stroke, diabetes, heart disease, and certain types of cancer. These conditions can be much more expensive than surgery, for they often involve hospitalization for weeks instead of days. Some health insurance provides coverage from the moment of admission, but other plans have a deductible period which is not covered.

When a diabetic undergoes surgery, it is not uncommon for his surgeon to call in a specialist or the patient's personal physician. In such cases the patient has two doctors taking care of him, and it is helpful if his insurance covers both their fees. This form of coverage is called concurrent care, and is especially necessary for the diabetic.

Another important aspect of health insurance for the diabetic is determining how much coverage to purchase. The policy which pays for every small expense, every visit to the doctor's office, every injection, is likely to be inadequate for meeting large expenses. Depending on the individual diabetic's physical condition and financial resources, he is often wiser to pay the small expenses out of his own pocket and get a health insurance plan that will completely cover major illness. Also, the patient should keep in mind that once he is flat on his back in the hospital, his family is going to have to worry about paying his medical and hospital bills. Therefore, he should consider the over-all economic structure of his family rather than only how much he can afford to pay this year in premiums. Once illness strikes, it is too late for a person to improve his own insurance coverage.

It is now possible for patients over sixty-five to take advantage of various federal and state programs which provide medical and hospital coverage. Local Social Security offices and state health agencies can provide specific details.

Health insurance is no longer restricted to only those who are employed by major firms, but rather it is available at reduced rates through almost any group such as a club or a trade union, as long as the group was founded for a purpose other than obtaining insurance.

DENTAL PROBLEMS

Dryness of the mouth is one of the first symptoms of diabetes, and patients who have had diabetes for many years sometimes complain of enlarged tongues with indentations around the edges. Dentists have noted that uncontrolled diabetes is associated with a marked increase in dental cavities, due perhaps to increased blood sugar levels and the diminished flow of saliva during the uncontrolled stages of the disease. Gum disease is also unusually prominent in diabetics.

Dental infection is quite serious, for an abscessed tooth or gum infection can throw the diabetes out of control, especially in those patients who respond poorly to stress. As the diabetes skids out of control, the dental condition worsens, and the vicious cycle can continue until the patient ends up in a diabetic coma. Care of the teeth is essential, for each time a tooth must be extracted or even drilled, the diabetic faces a potentially dangerous situation.

Close cooperation between physician and dentist is helpful, especially when a diabetic needs extensive dental work or extractions. Generally, all dental surgery, including extractions, should be delayed until after the diabetes is brought under good control. Naturally, there are times when this is not possible—when, for example, an abscess must be drained immediately. However, the better controlled the diabetes, the better the prognosis for extensive dental work.

When anesthesia is required, a local (a drug which deadens the nerves only in the immediate area of the operation, such as the jaw) is preferable to a general (one which produces unconsciousness). A diabetic should discuss his disease with his dentist, and should suggest a consultation between dentist and physician in the case of any abnormal dental problems.

CHAPTER 10

Have Diabetes,
Can Travel

Travel presents no particular problem to the diabetic, even those with insulin-dependent diabetes. Insulin need not be refrigerated as long as the temperature stays below 90 degrees Fahrenheit. Disposable syringes and needles, which were discussed earlier, eliminate the need for daily sterilization while traveling. Also insulin can be taken conveniently in the washroom of a plane or train or other convenient spot. If the temperature starts to climb above 90 degrees, it is helpful to place the insulin bottles inside either a thermos bottle or an insulated bag filled with cool water.

Ocean travel is no problem, since most passenger ships are equipped with adequate refrigeration for insulin storage. Even sailing is permitted, as long as the diabetic keeps the disease well controlled, tests his urine for sugar and acetone, and includes at least one companion who knows how to counteract insulin shock or acidosis.

Even though a diabetic may be able to obtain insulin in almost all countries, it is wiser to take along an adequate supply of insulin for the whole trip so that he is sure of having at his disposal the exact type of insulin he needs. This also is true for the oral drugs. There are some different sulfonylurea and biguanide drugs on the market in Europe, and their duration and mode of action may be different from or the same as the American-made drugs. To avoid confusion, it is best to take along a complete supply of the drugs.

The diagnostic material used for the urine tests are available, but may be difficult to find when needed. Therefore, to be safe, take along an ample supply.

The disposable insulin syringes and needles and foil-covered alcohol sponges are very convenient to have while traveling. These plastic syringes are also unbreakable.

Because diarrhea is a frequent pest while traveling in strange countries, due to the water or different foods, it is wise to ask the doctor for some medicine to control diarrhea.

Insulin-dependent diabetics should ask their physicians for explanatory letters to get them through foreign customs with a minimum of delay. This is necessary because customs officers might regard needles, syringes, and vials of insulin as indicative that the diabetic is really a narcotic addict. A brief note from a physician on his letterhead or prescription blank is usually sufficient to ward off the attentions of inspectors.

Before leaving this country, the diabetic should get from his doctor or from the American Diabetes Association* a list of diabetes associations in countries he plans to visit. Then, should his diabetes slip out of control, he can promptly get the name of a knowledgeable physician or clinic where he can be treated.

Should he find himself in trouble in a country

* 18 E. 48th St., New York, N.Y. 10017.

where there is no diabetes association or where he cannot speak the native language, a diabetic should contact the U.S. embassy for names of English-speaking physicians.

CHAPTER 11

Hypoglycemia: Low Concentrations of Sugar in the Blood

Hypoglycemia, which means low concentrations of sugar in the blood, is the opposite of diabetes, which is characterized by high blood sugar levels. Thus, the dangerously high blood sugars of overweight diabetics are lowered with the oral hypoglycemic drugs. Although hypoglycemia frequently precedes diabetes, it may also be a complete disease in its own right. It has full-blown symptoms and is difficult to diagnose because its symptoms resemble many other conditions.

There are two basic types of hypoglycemia, organic and functional. Organic hypoglycemia is caused by too much insulin in the bloodstream; an overdose of injected insulin can throw a diabetic into a state of hypoglycemia. Most of the time, however, organic hypoglycemia is a result of an internal defect, such as a disorder of the liver or the pituitary or adrenal glands, or a tumor on the brain or in the abdomen. Any such defect causes the pancreas to produce too much insulin.

The other basic category of the disease is functional hypoglycemia, for which no specific physical cause has been discovered. Nervousness, stress, depression, or severe prolonged muscular exertion often seem to be the culprits.

The symptoms of hypoglycemia are more numerous than for any other illness, because sugar—converted to glucose—is the body's fuel, and any disease that saps this energy will affect every part of the body. Hypoglycemia is often diagnosed as something else, for its symptoms can be almost identical with those of migraine headaches, ulcers, heart disease, or mental disturbances.

The principal victim of hypoglycemia is the brain, for it is the one organ which depends exclusively on blood sugar for food and oxygen. Other parts of the body can survive temporary sugar shortages by deriving energy from proteins and fats, but not the brain. Thus, any shortage of sugar starves the brain and results in improper functioning of the central nervous system, which coordinates and transmits brain impulses to muscles and bones. Disruption of the central nervous system and the body's metabolism can touch off numerous mental, emotional, and physical disorders. Also, oxygen shortage is the straightest path to irreversible brain damage and death.

Functional hypoglycemia is the more common but less serious of the two forms of the disease, for it is often transitory and immediately reversible. Many otherwise healthy individuals develop it because of a crash diet, strenuous exercise, lack of sleep, or often skipping meals. Do-it-yourself weight reduction is one of the more common causes of hypoglycemia, especially when the reducer tries to peel off pounds by simply not eating. Common symptoms of functional hypoglycemia include faintness, weakness, trembling, heart palpitations, profuse sweating, hunger, and nervousness. More severe symptoms are throbbing headache, confusion, visual disturbances, paralysis, staggering, and personality changes. Occasionally hypoglycemia will cause marked fatigue leading to unconsciousness, convulsive seizures, and coma. Although these last symptoms are the most serious, all the manifestations of hypoglycemia can be blamed on a lack of sugar in the blood supply feeding the brain.

The precise causes of these symptoms can usually be traced to some insufficiency in the endocrine glands which manufacture hormones that elevate blood sugar. And in some cases excess insulin is triggered by emotional excitement or tension. Such persons usually have highly sensitive pancreases which react also to stimulants such as excessive caffeine or nicotine, which cause excess insulin to pour into the bloodstream. Therefore, persons who experience any of the symptoms of hypoglycemia during excitement or tension should be particularly careful about the use of stimulants.

Although overweight is often a sign of diabetes, porky patients can also develop hypoglycemia. A low level of sugar in the blood can cause a craving for food, even an hour after a full meal. For this reason, a pre-dieting physical checkup is essential, but it should also include a blood sugar test. Hypoglycemia has foiled many well-planned and faithfully executed reducing programs, for when the body lacks fuel, it is almost impossible to get rid of body fat by limiting food consumption. Simultaneous treatment of overweight and low blood sugar creates no conflict, for the diets are similar—high in protein, low in starches and sugars and fats. A hypoglycemic patient who is not overweight need not worry about fats, which are, along with protein, absorbed more slowly than carbohydrate and do not produce a rush of insulin. Also, fats and protein are better than carbohydrate to appease the appetite, for they are slow-burning.

Therapy for hypoglycemia is quite simple, but it must be conducted under a physician's guidance to make sure that other organs of the body are not affected. In addition to diet, the hypoglycemic patient is urged to feed himself frequently. Six to eight small meals per day are better for him than three full meals. This maintains an even blood sugar level, and the pancreas is not overworked by peak loads of food. Because they are small, the frequent feedings do not lead to weight gain, although sometimes a vitamin supplement or tranquilizer may be prescribed, especially if tension tends to aggravate the hypoglycemia.

As more is learned about hypoglycemia and diabetes, certain relationships can occasionally be seen. For example, certain patients who show symptoms of functional hypoglycemia really have early diabetes. They maintain their hypoglycemia for a time, but diabetes, usually Type B or AB, but sometimes Type A, then sets in. Early treatment of the diabetes is difficult, for oral hypoglycemic drugs may worsen the hypoglycemia symptoms. Instead, treatment consists of the frequent feedings and a diet low in carbohydrate, high in protein, and moderate in fats.

Occasionally a patient will show symptoms of hypoglycemia (fatigue, nervousness, dizziness, cold sweat, etc.) but turn out to be a hyperventilator—that is, one who breathes too deeply and rapidly. This floods the brain with too much oxygen, and although the effect is just the opposite of hypoglycemia, the symptoms are similar, but this condition is called hyperventilation.

A dangerous form of the disease is alcohol-induced hypoglycemia. This can lead to coma following prolonged drinking during which the person's diet has been inadequate. Although little is known about this syndrome, it certainly is not caused by a defect of a body organ, nor is it restricted to chronic alcoholics.

Hypoglycemia is popular with the self-diagnosing crowd, for its symptoms are sufficiently common that the martini-drinking executive who is jittery and irritable assumes he has it, as does the plant foreman who suffers periodic hunger pangs. Self-diagnosis as such is harmless, if it leads the patient to his physician for confirmation. It becomes dangerous, however, when self-diagnosis leads to self-treatment, especially in the dieting. Many unknown hypoglycemics have battled heroically for years to take off weight, but they were unsuccessful. This alone should discourage the self-diagnoser against self-treatment.

PART V

The Future of
Diabetes

By 1970 the diabetic population in the United States will be four million. And there is little doubt that these figures will continue to expand throughout the rest of the twentieth century. (See Figure 9.) No immediate cure for diabetes is in sight, although one could conceivably be developed in a few years, once the basic causes of the disease are known.

Basic research is still sniffing at the heels of the defect responsible for diabetes, attempting to discover the flaw by studying its mechanisms and effects. One area of intense interest is the structure and function of the insulin molecule. This has been minutely mapped, revealing there are two parts to the insulin molecule, the "A-chain" and the "B-chain." Classification of the basic properties of the insulin molecule represents the first step toward synthesis and development of synthetic insulin. It remains only for the biochemists to combine the A-chain and B-chain to be able to make synthetic insulin. Synthetic insulin may mean a smoother-working, prolonged insulin, requiring only one injection a day for almost all insulin-dependent patients. Those patients who now have to take a special insulin made only from beef because they are allergic to pork could probably take synthetic insulin (insulin today is made from beef insulin or a combination of beef and pork insulin). It is doubtful, however, that diabetics will be able to take synthetic insulin orally, because the enzymes in the small intestine inactivate it.

There are probably two forms of circulating insulin, bound and free. The free form is active on muscle and fat tissue, but the bound form is inactive on muscle and selectively active on fat tissue. The precise nature of bound (or inactivated) insulin is

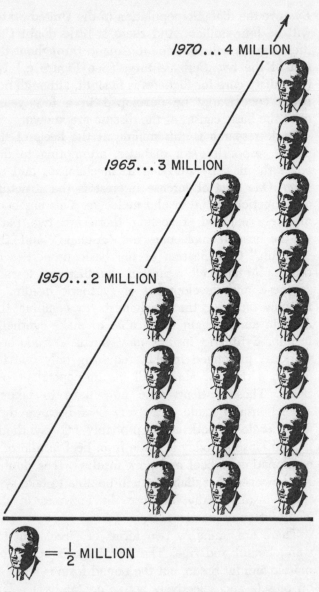

1970... 4 MILLION

1965... 3 MILLION

1950... 2 MILLION

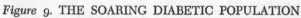 = ½ MILLION

Figure 9. THE SOARING DIABETIC POPULATION

still unknown. Some investigators think it may be a reserve supply which normal persons convert to the active form to maintain normal blood sugar levels. Also, it is suspected that a physiological defect of diabetes affects the binding and activating behavior of insulin and produces the symptoms of diabetes.

Another realm of investigation is concerned with the possibility that insulin may be antagonized or neutralized by antibodies so that the function of the insulin is inefficient—even though insulin production may be adequate.

Also under study is the role of glucagon, a hormone produced by the alpha cells of the pancreas (the beta cells release insulin). The function of glucagon appears to be to elevate the blood sugar level during times of need, which is precisely the opposite of insulin. Glucagon does this by releasing sugar that has been stored in the liver so that it gets into the bloodstream and can be used by the tissues. However, in an occasional instance it may be possible that an oversupply of glucagon could increase the blood sugar levels to the point where diabetes is mimicked or actually touched off.

Enzymes are the chemical foremen of the human factory, scurrying about throwing switches, releasing substances, and transforming, uniting, separating, breaking down, and reassembling molecules. Thus enzymes are unquestionably involved in the diabetic phenomenon, and research into the exciting possibilities is just beginning. If certain basic molecular activities could be understood in relation to how enzymes influence them, not only would the riddle of diabetes be solved, but specific enzyme inhibitors might then be developed to alter the diabetic state.

PRE-DIABETES

The electron microscope (which magnifies objects in excess of 100,000 times) has provided a method for determining the presence of diabetes long before it manifests itself through symptoms. Electron microscopic examination of ear lobe tissue in potential diabetics shows certain changes long before the disease appears to be present. Also, such examination has shown the capillaries, the tiniest blood vessels, to be abnormal, which might shed light on the atherosclerosis and degeneration of blood vessels which seems to be so closely allied with diabetes. One major goal of present research into pre-diabetes is to develop a practical means for the identification of future diabetics. Some success has been obtained with certain variations on the glucose tolerance test, such as the cortisone glucose tolerance test, but this still reveals the true diabetes phase, rather than the pre-diabetes phase. While these new methods may hold promise of bringing the patient to treatment earlier, they actually uncover not true pre-diabetes but rather patients in the chemical phase of true diabetes. For research purposes, the surest screening method thus far found is a history of diabetes in both parents. Newer avenues of research will come from the growing recognition that there is such a state as pre-diabetes.

GENETICS

Diabetes itself is not hereditary, but a predisposition or a tendency to inherit the disease is. A genetic error which transmits certain hereditary traits is passed on from parent to child throughout the generations. Although this genetic aspect of diabetes is well known, it is poorly understood. Current research is trying to track down the gene which creates a receptive physiological climate for diabetes. Successful detection of the guilty gene could lead to correction of the error and prevention of or even cure for diabetes.

TRANSPLANTATION

Considerable publicity has accompanied the efforts of physicians and surgeons to transplant organs and tissue from one living creature to another, especially from human to human. Most of these attempts have failed because the body reacts vigorously against the foreign tissue and refuses to cooperate with it. Attempts to transplant the pancreas have been as unsuccessful as those involving other organs.

New knowledge about how the human body reacts to foreign tissue is increasing the likelihood that transplants one day will be not only possible but common. The future may see transplants of live pancreatic tissue containing some of the Islets of Langerhans that produce insulin.

The future of diabetes is hazy because there is so much promising work just getting started in previously unexplored areas. Progress toward the cure of the disease is likely to be made gradually over several years, not dramatically or overnight. However, this is the first time in history when diabetics can look forward to ultimate victory of science over their disease. Diabetes is still a dangerous, capricious disease, if uncontrolled, but its days of power are numbered.

APPENDIX A

Height and Weight
Tables

Normal Height—Weight, ½ to 20 Years

AGE	MALE		FEMALE	
	HEIGHT	WEIGHT	HEIGHT	WEIGHT
YEARS	INCHES	POUNDS	INCHES	POUNDS
½	26	17	26	16
1	29	21	29	20
2	33	26	33	25
3	36	31	36	30
4	39	35	39	34
5	42	38	41	37
6	45	43	44	43
7	47	50	47	47
8	49	55	49	54
9	51	61	51	60
10	53	67	53	67
11	55	75	55	74
12	57	81	57	82
13	59	90	60	94
14	62	103	62	105
15	64	112	63	112
16	66	126	64	117
17	67	133	64	122
18	68	138	65	124
19	69	138	65	126
20	69	139	65	126

Desirable Weights for Men and Women*
According to Height and Frame, Ages 25 and Over

HEIGHT (in shoes, 1-inch heels)		MEN Weight in Pounds (in indoor clothing)		
FEET	INCHES	SMALL FRAME	MEDIUM FRAME	LARGE FRAME
5	2	112–120	118–129	126–141
5	3	115–123	121–133	129–144
5	4	118–126	124–136	132–148
5	5	121–129	127–139	135–152
5	6	124–133	130–143	138–156
5	7	128–137	134–147	142–161
5	8	132–141	138–152	147–166
5	9	136–145	142–156	151–170
5	10	140–150	146–160	155–174
5	11	144–154	150–165	159–179
6	0	148–158	154–170	164–184
6	1	152–162	158–175	168–189
6	2	156–167	162–180	173–194
6	3	160–171	167–185	178–199
6	4	164–175	172–190	182–204

HEIGHT (in shoes, 2-inch heels)		WOMEN Weight in Pounds (in indoor clothing)		
FEET	INCHES	SMALL FRAME	MEDIUM FRAME	LARGE FRAME
4	10	92– 98	96–107	104–119
4	11	94–101	98–110	106–122
5	0	96–104	101–113	109–125
5	1	99–107	104–116	112–128
5	2	102–110	107–119	115–131
5	3	105–113	110–122	118–134
5	4	108–116	113–126	121–138
5	5	111–119	116–130	125–142
5	6	114–123	120–135	129–146
5	7	118–127	124–139	133–150
5	8	122–131	128–143	137–154
5	9	126–135	132–147	141–158
5	10	130–140	136–151	145–163
5	11	134–144	140–155	149–168
6	0	138–148	144–159	153–173

* Metropolitan Life Insurance Company: Statistical Bulletin, *40:3*, 1959.

APPENDIX B

Energy Equivalents
of Food Calories Expressed in
Minutes of Activity

| | | ACTIVITY | | | | |
FOOD	CALORIES	Walking*	Riding Bicycle†	Swimming‡	Running#	Reclining‖
		min.	min.	min.	min.	min.
Apple, large	101	19	12	9	5	78
Bacon, 2 strips	96	18	12	9	5	74
Banana, small	88	17	11	8	4	68
Beans, green, 1 c.	27	5	3	2	1	21
Beer, 1 glass	114	22	14	10	6	88
Bread and butter	78	15	10	7	4	60
Cake, 1/12, 2-layer	356	68	43	32	18	274
Carbonated beverage, 1 glass	106	20	13	9	5	82
Carrot, raw	42	8	5	4	2	32
Cereal, dry, 1/2 c., with milk and sugar	200	38	24	18	10	154
Cheese, Cheddar, 1 oz.	111	21	14	10	6	85
Cheese, cottage, 1 tbsp.	27	5	3	2	1	21
Chicken, fried, 1/2 breast	232	45	28	21	12	178

FOOD	CALORIES	Walking* min.	Riding Bicycle† min.	Swimming‡ min.	Running# min.	Reclining‖ min.
Chicken, "TV" dinner	542	104	66	48	28	417
Cookie, chocolate chip	51	10	6	5	3	39
Cookie, plain	15	3	2	1	1	12
Doughnut	151	29	18	13	8	116
Egg, boiled	77	15	9	7	4	59
Egg, fried	110	21	13	10	6	85
French dressing, 1 tbsp.	59	11	7	5	3	45
Gelatin, with cream	117	23	14	10	6	90
Halibut steak, ¼ lb.	205	39	25	18	11	158
Ham, 2 slices	167	32	20	15	9	128
Ice cream, ⅙ qt.	193	37	24	17	10	148
Ice cream soda	255	49	31	23	13	196
Ice milk, ⅙ qt.	144	28	18	13	7	111
Malted milk shake	502	97	61	45	26	386
Mayonnaise, 1 tbsp.	92	18	11	8	5	71
Milk, 1 glass	166	32	20	15	9	128
Milk, skim, 1 glass	81	16	10	7	4	62
Milk shake	421	81	51	38	22	324
Orange, medium	68	13	8	6	4	52
Orange juice, 1 glass	120	23	15	11	6	92
Pancake with syrup	124	24	15	11	6	95

FOOD	CALORIES	Walking* min.	Riding Bicycle† min.	Swimming‡ min.	Running# min.	Reclining‖ min.
Peach, medium	46	9	6	4	2	35
Peas, green, ½ c.	56	11	7	5	3	43
Pie, apple, ⅙	377	73	46	34	19	290
Pie, raisin, ⅙	437	84	53	39	23	336
Pizza, cheese, ⅛	180	35	22	16	9	138
Pork chop, loin	314	60	38	28	16	242
Potato chips, 1 serving	108	21	13	10	6	83
Sandwiches						
Club	590	113	72	53	30	454
Hamburger	350	67	43	31	18	269
Roast beef with gravy	430	83	52	38	22	331
Tuna fish salad	278	53	34	25	14	214
Sherbet, ⅙ qt.	177	34	22	16	9	136
Shrimp, French-fried	180	35	22	16	9	138
Spaghetti, 1 serving	396	76	48	35	20	305
Steak, T-bone	235	45	29	21	12	181
Strawberry shortcake	400	77	49	36	21	308

* Energy cost of walking for 70-kg. individual = 5.2 calories per minute at 3.5 m.p.h.
† Energy cost of riding bicycle = 8.2 calories per minute.
‡ Energy cost of swimming = 11.2 calories per minute.
# Energy cost of running = 19.4 calories per minute.
‖ Energy cost of reclining = 1.3 calories per minute.

From *Journal of the American Dietetic Association,* courtesy of Dr. Frank Konishi.

List of Foods
to Be Avoided

Sugar
Candy
Honey
Jam
Jelly
Fried, scalloped,
   or creamed
     foods

Beer, wine,
   or other
   alcoholic
   beverages
Marmalade
Syrups
Pie
Cake

Cookies
Pastries
Condensed Milk
Soft drinks
   (sweetened
   with sugar)
Candy-coated
   gum

Note: These are general prohibitions, subject to a physician's specific revisions. Some diabetics will be permitted to eat a small amount of sweets in regular daily doses, while others might be allowed to drink alcohol moderately. A diabetic's personal diet will be dictated by the severity of his disease, his body weight, physical health, amount of daily exercise, and emotional adjustment.

APPENDIX D

Oral

Hypoglycemic

Agents

CHEMICAL NAME	TRADE NAME	
	U.S.	Foreign
Acetohexamide	Dymelor	Dymelor
Butyl biguanide		DBV
Carbutamide		BZ-55
Chlorpropamide	Diabinese	Diabinese
Dimethyl biguanide		Glucophage
Phenformin	DBI	Insoral DBI
Tolbutamide	Orinase	Rastinon Artosin Mobenol

INDEX